"As a woman of a certain age, I can attest to the truths within these pages. Had I had access to Bobbi Linkemer's book, *How to Age with Grace*, before leaving professional life, I would have had a much smoother transition into my current circumstances. Planning for one's retirement is good. Extensive planning is better. Precisely focused planning for any endeavor is best."

—Nattalia Nealls, retired Academic Personnel Specialist,
University of California San Diego

"Bobbi is a brilliant writer and the best person to write this book. She brings decades of writing experience to this project, which is a great culmination of her life's work—writing and living her own best life in every decade. It's practical, well-researched, and brings a light touch to topics many of us want to avoid. We all love older adults right now, and we hope to be one eventually, so this book is a necessity for all of us!"

—The Rev. Linda Anderson-Little,
Northern Texas - Northern Louisiana Synod, ELCA, author of
Motherhood Calling: Experiencing God in Everyday Family Life

Lynne

It is so good to see you!
Thank you for your interest
You are aging with grace!

Bobbi

HOW TO AGE WITH GRACE

Living Your Best Life in Your 70s, 80s, and Beyond

Bobbi Linkemer

Bobbi Linkemer's books on writing include:

Write Your Book Now:
A handbook for writers, authors, and self-publishers

How to Write a Nonfiction Book:
From planning to promotion in 6 simple steps

Going Solo:
How to survive and thrive as a freelance writer

Words To Live By:
Reflections on the writing life from a 40-year veteran

Before You Write Your Book:
Ask yourself these 8 important questions

The Savvy Ghostwriter:
Confessions of an Invisible Author (an e-book)

How to Write an Online Course:
From concept to completion one step at a time (an e-book)

The Book of Five:
Everything authors need to know about nonfiction books

The Skillful Writer:
What separates the pros from the amateurs

The Prosperous Author:
The business side of writing books

HOW TO AGE WITH GRACE

Living Your Best Life in Your 70s, 80s, and Beyond

Bobbi Linkemer

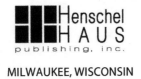

Henschel HAUS publishing, inc.

MILWAUKEE, WISCONSIN

Published by HenschelHAUS Publishing, Inc.
www.henschelHAUSbooks.com

ISBN: 978159598-803-4
E-ISBN: 978159598-804-1
Library of Congress Control Number: 2020952309

Cover and interior design by Peggy Nehmen: n-kreative.com

Printed in the United States of America.

Dedication

To my mother, who was

- Warm
- Open
- Loving
- Compassionate
- Generous
- Funny
- Witty
- Playful
- Smart
- Strong
- Wise
- Independent

And who knew the secret of aging with grace.

To my friend Ellen Brasunas, whose smile radiated *joie de vivre* and whose absence leaves a hole in the fabric of our lives. Ellen died of COVID two days after her ninety-sixth birthday.

*"Aging is not lost youth
but a new stage of
opportunity and strength."*

—Betty Friedan, author of
The Feminine Mystique and *The Fountain of Age*

Contents

FOREWORD

YOU ARE HOLDING IN YOUR HANDS the ultimate life-changing book that can have a positive impact on your life. This book speaks to all of us. We all age. Aging is inevitable, but are you prepared for what is to come? Just think for a moment. As you get older, what if you find yourself with no spouse by your side, no children to rely on, and no caregiver? How prepared would you be to spend your golden years with dignity and contentment?

The message in this book is powerful. Bobbi Linkemer draws from her own as well as others' valuable life experiences to offer us ten practical steps to help us successfully cope with our aging process.

We have become accustomed to a culture of going nonstop with work, family, activities, social life, and keeping up with the immediate demands of a fast-changing world. This book gives all of us a much-needed jolt to recognize and appreciate that aging will eventually catch up with everyone. When it does, will you be ready to face the reality of this inevitable phase of life? Will you be able to age gracefully and without stress?

There are many books out there that teach a lesson or two about aging, but this book is different. You are at once gripped by powerful, real-life stories that create a sense of urgency to do something. The decisions you make now can affect your life in the years to come, and planning now for the challenges you will face later as you near the end of your career or your life are the key take-home messages from this book.

While aging is inevitable, *how* you age and *how* you prepare yourself are within your control. This book should serve as a manifesto for how to age wisely and gracefully.

For those who accept the fact that life will not stay the same as you age, here is a way to understand and cope with the inevitable changes ahead. *How to Age with Grace* offers ways to respond to and embrace ten essential aspects of life that every one of us will face sooner or later.

Bhupendra O. Khatri, MD, FAAN
Medical Director of The Regional MS Center &
The Center for Neurological Disorders in Milwaukee, Wisconsin
Author of bestselling books, *Healing the Soul,* and *Healthcare 911,*
winner of three national awards.

PREFACE

I HAVE NOTICED THAT WHATEVER is going on in my life is reflected in my bookcases. There is a whole shelf devoted to Buddhism and mindfulness, another one with books for and about women, two shelves of books I have helped others write, one shelf for biographies and memoirs, parts of shelves for whatever I was researching at the time, one for books on health and fitness, and most recently, one that is rapidly filling up with books about aging. It doesn't take a genius to know that this latest topic is very much on my mind.

I have always seemed to read the right book at the right moment. In my forties, I read Gail Sheehy's *Passages*; in my fifties, *New Passages* and *The Silent Passage*. If I needed to be inspired by journalists and notable writers, I read books by Leslie Stahl, Linda Ellerbe, Gloria Steinem, and Anne Morrow Lindbergh. In my endless search for answers to life's big questions, I read my way through New Age, world religions, Judaism, and Native American spirituality. And now, as I celebrate milestone birthdays and struggle to overcome my existential fear of aging, I know that it is time to face it, to learn everything I can about it, and to accept it.

Once you pass your eightieth birthday, which I did four years ago, you are officially old. Even if nobody comes close to guessing your age, your body has been recording the passage of time from day one and knows exactly how old you are. If you are one of the fortunate few, you may still look and feel younger than your biological age. You may be full of energy, free of major maladies, mentally sharp, and highly productive.

If this describes you, I would thank your ancestors for the gift of good genes, as well as give yourself some credit for living well.

I don't mean to imply that those who do not fit this profile are aging poorly, are unhappy, or are sick. I belong to a writers' group where three of the members are in their nineties and still going strong. On the other hand, many of my peers who are far short of their nineties are living with ailments that go along with getting older. As each of us copes with our own aging process, it's worth noting that our population as a whole is also aging. In fact, the fastest-growing segment of adults in this country comprises those over eighty-five. In 2012, the United Nations estimated that there were 316,600 living centenarians worldwide.

As our numbers grow, so does the strain on our healthcare system and our adult children, who often find themselves trying to meet the needs of both their own children and their aging parents. Most of us do not reflect the stereotypical picture of old people living out their days in rocking chairs. On the contrary, the majority of people I know who are in their seventies, eighties, and nineties strive to retain as much of their independence as possible. They prefer to "age in place," as opposed to living with their children or in retirement facilities. They stay active and involved in life, are interesting and fun to be around, and continue to contribute their time and talents wherever possible.

Most of us are realistic about our current stage in life. We know where we are and what may lie ahead in the coming years. We know that if we want to have a say in how the rest of our lives unfold, we have important decisions to make. Facing the number and complexity of those decisions may seem overwhelming at first, but they don't all have to be made at once or alone. There is help available from our children and many other sources. But, ultimately, if our minds are working well, we are perfectly capable of meeting this challenge.

This book was born out of my own need to understand what those decisions are and to gather the necessary information to make them wisely. The more I talked to people and began to organize my thoughts, the more I realized that others could benefit from what I was learning. I am a big believer in lists, as nothing seems too big to tackle when it's in a simple list. Here was my list of topics to investigate:

1. Attitude
2. Living independently
3. Safety
4. Driving
5. Health
6. Retirement
7. Talking to adult children
8. Money
9. Friendships
10. End of life

As I launched this project, I planned to do a lot of research, including interviewing people who had something to say about each of the items in that list. I anticipated that I would talk to professionals in various related fields, people I knew and people I didn't know, and just about anyone who might add to my understanding of this subject matter. Then, of course, I would go the academic route through Internet searches, reference librarians, books by other authors, memoirs, and biographies.

I confess that this was not my customary way of attacking a new book. I usually have a clearer idea of content—an outline that is quite detailed. This time, however, I decided to trust the creative process and let the outline emerge more organically. I pictured the book being a combination of my own thoughts, the observations of others, and factual information I gathered along the way. Writing this way was a little like taking a trip without a GPS or map. The destination was not set in stone, and the route meandered. I knew it was a faith leap, but I was confident that the journey would be fascinating, and I would end up knowing a lot more than I knew when I started. I was right.

ACKNOWLEDGMENTS

Every book has its heroes (in this case, heroines), whose talent and skills bring an author's words to life. My heartfelt thanks to my heroines:

- Judy Mosbacher, my sister, my best friend, my editor
- Peggy Nehmen, who, once again, created the perfect book design
- Kira Henschel, who believed in this book enough to publish it
- Lesley DeMartini, whose meticulous editing enhanced my writing

And to all those who shared their wisdom and experience on *How to Age with Grace*:

- Roberta Balke
- Ellen Brasunas
- Eileen Carlson
- Benita Crook
- Joann Dyroff
- Robin Garnett
- Diana Gates
- Felicia Graber
- Jonathan Gordon
- Barbara Florio Graham
- Bill Hosner
- Andi and Pete Krehbiel
- Paul Lang
- Janell Nunn
- Alan Ranford
- Vicki Spraul
- Billie Teneau
- Monique Williams, MD

INTRODUCTION

AMERICA IS GOING GRAY. We see evidence all around us every day. The current growth of those aged sixty-five and older, driven by the large Baby Boom generation, is unprecedented in US history. Their number is **projected to nearly double** from 52 million in 2018 to 95 million by 2060, and their share of the total population will rise from 16 percent to 23 percent.

In less than two decades, the graying of America will be inescapable. Americans are having fewer children, and the Baby Boom of the 1950s and 1960s has yet to be repeated. Fewer babies and longer life expectancy equal a faster-aging country. And with that aging comes a whole host of unknowns, both for the country, which is ill-prepared to care for the increasing number of older people, and for the older people themselves. One of the unknowns is how the country will support its elders, with fewer young people than ever before paying into Social Security.

Older people are also dealing with unknowns, including the COVID-19 pandemic. In this stage of their lives, they find themselves in unfamiliar territory. To many seniors, it is a baffling maze. Finding answers to their questions often turns into a research project; in many cases, they don't even know what questions to ask.

That was my experience a few years ago when I pondered whether to stop driving, close my business, give up my cozy little condo, move to a retirement community, and live on less than the recommended amount of money I should have saved for my retirement. These were daunting questions, for sure. If I answered yes to any one of them, at least one aspect of my life would change dramatically. Part of me wasn't ready, but another part of me recognized the need to face my own aging process with clear eyes and an open mind.

On the very first topic—whether to give up my car—I had one aha moment after another. I could have written a book on that subject alone. I looked up statistics on Americans over sixty-five and found an abundance a of information.

According to the US Census Bureau, "The elderly population will more than double between now and the year 2050, to 80 million. By that time, as many as one in five Americans could be elderly. Most of this growth should occur between 2010 and 2030, when the 'Baby Boom' generation enters their elderly years. The 'oldest old'—those aged eighty-five and over—are the most rapidly growing elderly age group. Between 1960 and 1994, their numbers rose 274 percent from 3 million in 1994 to a projected 19 million in 2050."

In a 2016 article in *Forbes*, "The biggest story, of course, is the sheer number of aging Baby Boomers. By 2016, one of every seven Americans, or 49 million, had reached age sixty-five. By 2060, that number will double to 98 million Americans being at least sixty-five ... About 82,000 Americans were one hundred or older in 2016, and that number could increase ten-fold by mid-century."

Wouldn't most of those older people have many of the same questions I had? Would they know what clues to look for when it was time to retire, stop living alone or stop driving, and talk to their adult children about such painful subjects as preparing for death? Do they know what steps to take to keep themselves healthy and safe? Those were the questions that played over and over in my mind, and I felt sure I was not alone. Why not share what I was learning with a built-in audience of senior citizens who were in exactly the same place in life as I was? And so *How to Age with Grace: Living Your Best Life in Your 70s, 80s, and Beyond* began to take shape.

I knew I didn't want to write a memoir or an authoritative tome. I didn't want my perspective to be the only one expressed or to speak for my entire generation. And yet, I needed just a slice of each of those approaches to talk to other older adults in an accessible, conversational style. Thus this book became one part personal reflections on my own experience; one part insights, observations, and facts based on research; and one part interviews with experts in various fields and older people who are trying to live their best lives.

Millions of people have grown old since the beginning of time; yet, for each of us, aging is a singular experience. How well we handle the inevitable changes that come with this stage of life, what profound lessons we are able to apply to our own lives, and the wisdom we pass along to the next generation are the measures of grace we bring to our own aging process.

Here is what you can expect in the ten chapters that follow:

I. Seeing Clearly: *What is the best attitude to help you through the aging process?*
Coping with the inevitable changes of aging is never easy, but there will be fewer surprises if we know what to expect. While there is no doubt that modern medicine can do wonders to slow down or even reverse the natural erosion of body parts, we play a role in preventing the predictable effects of aging. The more we understand our own bodies, the better able we are to keep them functioning well into our later years. Of course, feeling positive about getting old is easier when age is respected and older people are valued more than they are in our youth-obsessed society. We may not be able to do much to change someone else's opinion, but if this is the image we have of ourselves, we can and must do something about it. What *we* need is a more positive, yet realistic, self-image—a new perception of who we are, what we are capable of, and what we can contribute to society. This is a choice—a choice we have the power

to make. We can choose to be miserable about each passing year and physical change, or we can try to adapt to the natural flow of life.

II. Going Solo: *Are you ready to stop living on your own?*

Who decides when it's time to reconsider your living arrangements—you or your family? When you realize that your health is failing or grocery shopping and cooking have become chores, it's obvious you could use some help. If you don't want to live with your children or move to a retirement community, you would probably prefer to "age in place"— to remain in your home, as long as you can do so safely. You have a significant role to play in staying as healthy and alert as possible for as long as possible. The biggest clue that you need help is when you find yourself falling. Falling is frightening, as well as an indication that your mobility has become more limited. This is the time to take an honest inventory of both your health and your home. For a physical problem, sometimes a simple examination is what you need for an accurate diagnosis and appropriate treatment. If your home is the problem, take a good look around so that you can identify potential hazards. You will be grateful for the time you spent eliminating the harmless-looking obstacles that could land you on the floor.

III. Getting Serious About Safety: *What does it take to accident-proof your surroundings?*

The most essential human need—beyond the necessity for air, water, and food—is to be safe. Anyone can slip on ice, miss a step walking down the stairs, trip over an unseen wire, or lose her balance. There are hidden hazards everywhere you look or, more accurately, where you don't look. The national survey on fear of crime, *The Figgie Report*, indicates that "four out of five Americans are afraid of being assaulted, robbed, raped, or murdered. Being constantly afraid may kill you faster than violence itself." This is particularly relevant to older people because an ongoing fear for your personal safety can systematically destroy brain cells, which accelerates the aging of your mind. Rather than give in to fear, become aware of potential dangers, make sensible plans for actions you can take, and then put an end to chronic worry about safety. For every potential danger you can think of, there are numerous preventive actions you can take to keep yourself safe, many of which you can do yourself. Information is power. The more you know about the risks involved, the better prepared you can be to deal with them.

IV. Turning in Your Car Keys: *When is the right time for you to stop driving?*

According to the AAA Foundation for Traffic Safety, by the year 2031, one in every five drivers in America will be sixty-five years of age or older. While our experience does not decline with age, some of the skills necessary for safe driving—vision, reflexes, flexibility, and hearing—do begin to deteriorate. I have heard it said that older people self-monitor, and when we realize we're having trouble doing something, we stop doing it. Why, then, do most people drive seven to ten years longer than they should? There is no set age for when people should stop driving, but important decisions, such as whether to stop, should be made based on knowing the facts. It is an irrefutable fact that people age seventy and older are more likely to crash than any other age group. And because older drivers are more fragile, they are also more likely to get hurt or die from these crashes. A few years ago, there would have been practically no options except cabs and begging rides. But now we have the miracle of Lyft, Uber, and such national organizations as Aging Ahead and ITN*Gateway*. You can give up your car and still get around. Such adjustments will take some getting used to, but then, change always does.

V. Staying Healthy: *What will it take to maintain your vigor and vitality?*

When we human beings age, inevitable changes take place in our bodies. Some of these changes are out of our control; they are simply part of being human. But we do have the power to slow down or even prevent some of the diseases and changes in how we look and feel. The more we understand about our own bodies and what they need, the better able we will be to live long and healthy lives. Scientific studies have revealed that the human body self-destructs as we age, but the speed at which it breaks down is up to us.

The opposite of early self-destruction is healthy aging. Technically, healthy aging is being free of disease, functioning at a high physical and cognitive level, and being socially engaged and productive. According to Dr. Andrew Weil, a well-known American doctor who promotes a holistic approach to medicine, "Although aging is an irreversible process, there are myriad things you can do to keep your mind and body in good working order through all phases of your life. Aging doesn't mean you have to get old in the process."

VI. Deciding to Retire: *How do you know when you're ready to stop working?*

If you are still struggling with whether to retire or keep working, answer the following questions as honestly as you can:

• *Can you afford to retire based on the money or investments you have?*
You should have at least 70 to 80 percent of your yearly salary saved for every year of retirement. If you made $100,000 a year when you were employed, you will need to earn $80,000 or 80 percent every year to retire at a comfortable level.

• *How much money will you need to live close to the lifestyle you are living now?*
If what you need is far more than what you have, consider postponing retirement for a year or two.

• *How healthy are you and your spouse, if you have one?*

If you are in excellent health and your family has longevity genes, keep working if you want to.

• *Do you and your spouse picture your retirement years in the same way?*
If not, you will need talk about this and resolve your differences. When you're married, you have to think of retirement as a team sport.

• *How much do you need to cover your healthcare now and in the foreseeable future?*
If you are a sixty-five-year-old couple, who retired in 2020, you will need close to $400,000 to cover healthcare expenses, including Medicare Parts B and D. Dental care is not covered by original Medicare.

• *Are you planning to live on your Social Security alone?*
Twenty-three percent of married retirees and 43 percent of single retirees count on Social Security for 90 percent or more of their monthly income. So, it can be done.

VII. Talking to Your (Adult) Children: *Can you (and they) face the tough questions?*
What is the magic age when we are considered old and in need of constant monitoring and care? Our kids may be stressed out over feeling obligated to help us, but it is equally stressful for us to find ourselves the recipients of help we didn't think we needed and to feel our independence slipping away. Being independent means that we will be able to go through challenging life situations, as we always have, without depending on our children to help us cope. *The more independent we are, the greater our self-confidence and self-esteem will be.*

Another difficult subject, especially for our adult children, is the need to put our affairs in order before the end of our lives. In the midst of coping with the medical, emotional, psychological, and spiritual challenges of having a serious illness, we or our children will also have to manage mundane logistical details. Of course, the subject of our death will be hard for our children to talk about calmly and rationally. So, how we approach the subject and take our children's feelings into account will make all the difference in how the conversation goes.

VIII. Figuring Out Your Finances: *Are you prepared to retire?*
The one subject no senior citizen can afford to ignore is also the one subject many of us find uncomfortable to discuss: money. At one end of the spectrum are those who have thought through and planned every aspect of their retirement; at the other end are those who are retiring on a wing and prayer, with little to no planning and limited financial resources. For this group, the subject is a particularly tough one, because not only are they unprepared, often they don't know what questions to ask or where to find the answers. At any time of one's life, money can be a confusing and emotional topic. When money is tight and today's bills are piling up, preparing for retirement isn't even on the radar.

By 2030, more than seventy million Baby Boomers will be sixty-five or older. In the meantime, according to the *Washington Post*, "Each day, ten thousand retire and begin receiving Medicare and Social Security benefits. Unfortunately, the vast majority will not have sufficient savings to retire full-time at sixty-five with their pre-retirement standard of living."

IX. Building Your Support System: *How will you build and maintain your social circle?*
We need friends all our lives but never more than in our later years. Friends become increasingly important to health and happiness as people age. Having strong social bonds helps us live longer, boosts our immune systems, decreases high blood pressure, and allows us to enjoy a more meaningful life. Having secure friendships can help to reduce stress, chronic pain, and the risk of heart disease—all good reasons to

make friends. It isn't only important to have friends, but the quality of those friendships matters just as much.

Life is unpredictable, especially as we grow older. When we hit a rough patch, we need those who will understand what we are going through—or at least be able to listen to us as we vent. We need this because giving and receiving support from others is a basic human need; because having a support system leads to higher levels of well-being, better coping skills, and a longer and healthier life; and because it reduces depression and anxiety. Once you have made some new friends, you must keep those friendships alive and thriving.

X. Facing End-of-Life Choices: *How do you make your wishes known and fulfilled?*

Dying is inevitable, and knowing that, logic suggests that we should be better prepared when it comes. Preparation means facing reality and taking the necessary steps to let those who are close to us know what we hope for in our final days. Many people wait until they are terminally ill or in a life-threatening situation before they confront end-of-life decisions and plans. Of course, facing them is never easy, but we must do so while we are still thinking clearly and able to articulate our desires.

Some of the powerful emotions we can expect to have include fear, anger, guilt, regret, grief, anxiety, depression, and loneliness. Human beings need meaning in our lives. We are hardwired to seek a reason for being here and for what has happened to us along the way. As I mention in Chapter VII: "Talking to Your Adult Children," the essential documents are a will, advanced directives or a living will, a durable power of attorney for healthcare, and your preferences about your funeral and/or memorial service. Filling out those important documents requires introspection and self-reflection.

The average life expectancy in the United States is seventy-nine. There are some aspects of reaching that age or beyond that are out of our control, such as gender, genetics, access to healthcare, and crime rates. But, according to *Disabled World*, the rest is due to such factors as hygiene, diet and nutrition, exercise, and lifestyle, which are within our control and can be modified by changing our behavior. The one thing we can control completely it is our *attitude* (see Chapter I: "Seeing Clearly"), which has a profound effect on both the quantity of our years and the quality of our habits (www.disabled-world.com, 3/3/2019).

I. SEEING CLEARLY

*What is the best attitude to help you
through the aging process?*

IN MANY PARTS OF THE WORLD, the elderly are treated with respect—even reverence—for the experience and wisdom they have accumulated during their lifetimes. Unfortunately, in our Western society, if we revere anything, it is youth, not age. This is regrettable, since our population is aging at warp speed; one of the fastest-growing segments comprises those who are eighty-five or older. This group is projected to more than double from 6.4 million in 2016 to 14.6 million in 2040—a 129 percent increase.

Knowing how one's attitude colors everything from personality to longevity, I began this book in an effort to understand my not-quite-positive attitude towards my own aging and, if possible, change it.

Fixing What We Can See

Most studies on this subject conclude that older people are happier and healthier than ever before—certainly much happier than when we were middle-aged. Many of us see ourselves as independent, vital, and active, but others may not share that image. If we have wrinkled skin or gray hair, it stands to reason we must be old—so we go on diets, color our hair, and join Zumba classes. The result of this effort and expense is that we look better than ever, but beneath the surface, physical and emotional changes are taking place whether they are obvious or not.

Coping with these inevitable changes is never easy, but taking some of the mystery out of what is happening may help. For one thing, there will be fewer surprises if we know what to expect; for another, we can prevent, or at least forestall, some of these changes by practicing good health habits.

The Changes We Can't See

Here's what we should know about what happens to our bodies as we age. It's not necessarily a cheerful picture, but it's a natural part of life—and in almost all cases, there are things we can do to ameliorate the changes. Our bones become thinner and weaker, especially in post-menopausal women, who are at risk of osteoporosis and potentially dangerous falls. Our reflexes, memory, the rate our hearts pump blood, digestion, and metabolism all slow down. Our senses, such as smell, taste, touch, vision, and hearing, diminish. Plaques and tangles form in the brain, which can damage our brains and nerve cells and possibly lead to dementia. Our skin begins to wrinkle and lose its elasticity. Post-menopausal women experience vaginal dryness or lack of lubrication, while men encounter erectile dysfunction. And, finally, stress and grief due to the loss of people we love, our purpose in life when we are no longer working, and the empty nest when our children leave home take their toll. If we don't learn to manage these stressors effectively, we will be more vulnerable to physical illness.

That is a daunting list, to be sure. It's no wonder so many of us dread the years ahead as if we are little more than crumbling machines that are breaking down one nut and bolt at a time.

Understanding Our Bodies

But we are not machines, and while there's no doubt that modern medicine can do wonders to slow down or even reverse the natural erosion of body parts, we play a role in preventing the predictable effects of aging. The more we understand our own bodies, the better able we are to keep them functioning well into our later years.

Let's face it: We are one of many animal species, and like all the rest, we were never intended to live forever. The big difference between humans and other species is that we have awareness of ourselves and our situations, choices about what to do to change what can be changed, and the ability to act on them. We are not omnipotent; we can't change everything, such as our heredity, but neither are we helpless. There are many things we can do to make aging more pleasant and even vibrant. (For much more on this subject, see Understanding the Changes that Come with Age in Chapter V: Staying Healthy.)

Life in *The Blue Zones*

Books and studies abound about people in their advanced years running marathons, climbing mountains, and leaving younger competitors in the dust. One book that is getting a lot of attention and has spawned an industry is *The Blue Zones, Second Edition: 9 Lessons for Living Longer From the People Who've Lived the Longest* by Dan Buettner. The term "blue zones" refers to geographic areas throughout the world in which people have low rates of chronic disease and live longer than anywhere else.

According to the Amazon blurb, "A healthy life is no accident. It begins with good genes, but it also depends on good habits. If we adopt the right lifestyle, experts say, chances are we can add decades to our lives." It appears to be exactly what the people in the Blue Zones have done. By practicing good habits and the right lifestyle, they have extended their lives beyond their hundredth birthdays.

Buettner traveled the world seeking the secrets of longevity through stories and interviews with some of the most remarkable, happy, and healthy centurions on the planet. His conclusion: "It's no coincidence that the way they eat, interact with each other, shed stress, heal themselves, avoid disease, and view their world yield them more good years of life."

In Blue Zones, which are all over the world, people respect the elderly, and the prevailing attitude is happiness. While this may sound like a fairy tale, it is grounded in years of research, interviews, and hard science. Of course, genetics and the environment play important roles, but the key seems to be lifestyle.

The Invisible Older Woman

It's easier to feel positive about getting old when age is respected, and older people are valued, which is not the case in our youth-obsessed society. Best-selling author Betty Friedan, in her 1993 book, *The Fountain of Age*, lamented that older women are becoming invisible in many settings, including executive positions in business, top roles in movies, and placement in magazine advertising. When I read that part of Friedan's book twenty-six years ago, I was sure she was exaggerating, but from my present vantage point, I have changed my mind. On many occasions in recent years, I have felt not only unseen but also irrelevant.

Is this how the world sees, or doesn't see, "women of a certain age," or is this the way we see ourselves? If this is truly the world's perception, we may not be able to do much to change someone else's opinion. On the other hand, if this is the image we have of ourselves, we can and must do something about it. Buying into this inaccurate, demeaning stereotype is a self-inflicted wound. It isn't true, it isn't healthy, and it certainly isn't a way to age with grace.

What *is* healthy is a more positive, yet realistic, self-image—a new perception of who we are, what we are capable of, and what we can contribute to society. Let me be clear: I am *not* Pollyanna, who could find the silver lining in the darkest cloud. In fact, as I mentioned earlier, my attitude about aging could often use a makeover, and I know I am not alone in admitting that. But knowing I need an attitude adjustment, and then developing one, will not be any easier than losing a hundred pounds. There is little difference between being a hundred pounds overweight and nurturing a negative, self-destructive picture of yourself. Both will make you sick.

The Mind-Body Connection

The relationship between the mind and body is believed to have first been studied by the philosopher, René Descartes, so it is hardly new. But it's important to understand how the mind and body work together if you really want to change something as deeply ingrained as your view of yourself. The mind-body connection simply means that your thoughts, feelings, beliefs, and attitudes can positively or negatively affect your biological functioning. In other words, your mind can affect how healthy your body is. That simple statement can change your life.

How is that possible? According to Dr. James Gordon, founder of the Center for Mind-Body Medicine at the University of Minnesota, "The brain and peripheral nervous system, the endocrine and immune systems, all the organs of our body, and indeed, all the emotional responses we have, share a common chemical language and are constantly communicating with one another."

It is no stretch to see how this applies to the power of our attitudes and the need to change their adverse effect on our health. The question, of course, is how do we do that? There are hundreds of ideas, ranging from trying a new hobby to taking up tennis. If we followed even half of them, we would be busy all the time.

Much of what I've said so far applies to many of us in our age group, but let's make the conversation a little more personal. Let's talk about how all of this applies to *you*. I suggest that before you get busy *doing* things to slow down the aging process, begin by *accepting the changes that are happening* instead of *trying to resist them*. Getting old is inevitable. Our bodies change, our loved ones die, the world we once knew no longer exists. You can kick and scream and rail at fate, but this will change nothing except the state of your health. The only thing you can change is your response to what life throws at you. Since the issue here is getting older, and you can't reverse it or stop it from happening, your only alternative is to accept reality.

Making Wise Choices

This is a choice—a choice you have the power to make. You can choose to be miserable about each passing year and physical change, or you can try to adapt to the natural flow of life. Once you've made that choice, you can begin to consider some of the actions you can take to reawaken the vitality that has taken a time out.

Of all the things you have to do to change your attitude and live your seventies, eighties, and beyond with grace, you have just done the hardest one. Once you accept that you are in a perfectly natural stage of life, the next step is to ask yourself what you need to be happy. When I look at my own life, I know I need people—but not just any people. I need my family and my circle of friends. This is my support system in good times and bad. The saying that "no man is an island" is true. You cannot lock yourself up in your house and become a recluse. You need people almost as much as you need air.

Human beings are social animals. The third level of Maslow's hierarchy of needs is love and belonging. I am fortunate to be very close to my family, but I know that is not true of everyone. If your family is not your support system or is scattered around the country, don't despair. They say you can't choose your relatives, but you can choose your friends. So, do it. But choose them carefully because, over time, those friends can become the family you create.

Try to spend time with at least one person every day. The time doesn't have to be long and involved. It can be as simple as taking a walk, running into each other at the grocery store or the gym, or something more structured, such as signing up for class together. If you are feeling lonely or blue, that's all the more reason to seek someone to talk to. It doesn't have to be your best friend or a long conversation. A chat with the librarian at your local library or one of your neighbors walking her dog might suffice.

Without a doubt, the one nonnegotiable item on your list should be physical exercise. Humans were meant to move, no matter our age. As a matter of fact, the older we are, the more important it is to keep moving. If we don't maintain our flexibility and balance, strengthen our muscles, and increase our endurance, we are putting ourselves at risk. Staying physically active reduces the odds of developing heart disease, stroke, and diabetes; lowers your blood pressure; prevents depression; and helps you lose weight.

It's hardly a news flash that regular aerobic exercise keeps our hearts and lungs healthy, our bones strong, and our minds sharp. In fact, one of the greatest benefits of exercise is its effect on our brains. Exercise reduces the brain fog that comes with age, protects memory and thinking skills, improves mood and sleep, and reduces stress. Aerobic and resistance training helps relieve chronic pain from arthritis and lower-back problems, boosts your immune system and improves your sleep, helps reverse bone loss, lowers your blood pressure, enhances your balance, strengthens your arms and back, and as an added bonus, increases your self-confidence.

By now, you should be convinced that exercise can bring energy and enthusiasm to your later years. The next step is to tie up the laces of your workout shoes and get moving. This may be the most important thing you ever do for yourself.

The Need for Support

The feelings you're grappling with are hardly unique. If you talk to your friends, you know this. As a matter of fact, talking to your friends is a wonderful way to cope with whatever is on your mind. Consider inviting some of them over for coffee, and just sit around and talk. You or someone else in the group can hold this type of informal get together whenever you choose. Before you realize it, you will have formed a support group of other people who are coping with the challenges of the aging process just as you are. Support groups are powerful.

Most of us remember the consciousness-raising groups we belonged to in the early 1970s when we first became aware of something called the Women's Movement. Those groups and the results they produced changed many of our lives. We went to work or back to school. We started our own businesses. We explored long-forgotten talents and ambitions. And we changed the culture. Society began to take women seriously.

Wouldn't it be wonderful if we could replicate that success when it comes to the way society views older people? What would it take to make that happen? Could our little support groups accomplish what those consciousness-raising groups did so many years ago? What an accomplishment it would be if we could once again change the culture and have society begin to take the elderly seriously.

Add to Your To-Do List

While we are waiting to change the world, there are still plenty of things to do that will have a positive effect on your attitude about growing older. If you are mobile and perhaps still driving, explore places in your city you have never been to, such as a museum, an art gallery, concerts in the park, or historic homes you always meant to visit. Ask a friend with similar interests to join you, and make it a mini adventure.

Have you abandoned activities and hobbies you used to enjoy, such as riding a bike, golfing, playing the piano, baking, painting, or writing in a journal? Why not try a few of them again? In 1990, Italian-born psychologist Mihaly Csikszentmihalyi introduced the concept of *Flow: The Psychology of Optimal Experience*, which beautifully describes the state of mind in which people are so involved in an activity that nothing else seems to matter. They become so focused on what they're doing that they lose track of time and forget to move. It's hard to find the right words to describe how you feel when you're in flow—trance-like, hypnotic, in the zone, meditative. One thing is for sure: you don't feel old.

I could go on and on about all the things you can do to explore, learn, and do. The list is as long as your imagination. You could travel to some destination you want to see, which could be as close as across the river or as far away as across the ocean, depending on your finances and ability to travel.

You could start a book club, learn a new language, take a course in your local university's lifelong learning program, volunteer at a hospital or for some organization you want to support, join a writing group, or write a memoir. And, finally, you could become one of the 35 million Americans who do some form of meditation. Few things I can think of will release the power of your attitude as profoundly as meditation.

I want to leave you with one last thought that is perhaps the most important of all of the activities I have suggested. You have accomplished many things in your life so far. Perhaps you have raised a family or built a successful career. Maybe you have created art or written books, volunteered at a hospital, been a docent at a museum, taught school, been active in your church or synagogue, worked in the food pantry, or contributed to your community in other ways. You may still be involved in many of these activities, or you may have felt it was time to take a break. The point is that you have done all these things and had an impact on many people. Just because you are no longer doing them does not in any way diminish their value.

I have a friend who raised two children, went back to school, earned her PhD, and wrote the psychology book that is required reading in many school psychology classes across the country. It took her many years to write that book, which will be read by countless students in the future. While it was hardly her only achievement in life, it was certainly one of the most significant. No matter what else she accomplishes in the years to come, that book will always be a permanent reminder of something of value she created. She called it her *monument*—the one thing she has done that no one can ever undo or take away.

At times when she is doubting her value or feeling invisible, it is important for my friend, as it is for all of us in such moments, to take an inventory of what we have produced in our lives. Sometimes that is difficult to do when your accomplishments are intangible. Not everyone can hold a book in her hands as a reminder that this is something she wrote. There are so many things you have done in your life, so many ways that you have brightened someone's day or helped in some way that you may not have even realized. These moments are all evidence of a life well lived—a life of "monuments" to be proud of.

Roberta Balke
A Lifelong Optimist

Roberta Balke has always been an upbeat, positive person. She attended the University of Illinois for two years, left to get married, raised four children, and then returned to school to continue her interrupted education. Along the way, she earned a BA in psychology and an MA in counseling and psychology at Governors State University. She retired from her position as assistant dean of Moraine Valley Community College in 1999. At eighty-three, Roberta is a lifelong learner who has discovered CSPAN 3 and YouTube as sources of continuing education.

I think I was born optimistic, or maybe it was because of growing up in an environment that was negative. I always looked at the cup as half full. When my daughter would suggest going somewhere for the weekend, I never even hesitated. I always said, "Let's go. I'm in." When we were on the road, if we hit a lot of traffic, our thing would be to see how we could make lemonade out of lemons. So, that became my mantra.

Perseverance is probably my greatest strength. I may not have had all the talents I would have liked, but I was always able to put one foot in front of the other and move forward. I do know you need to develop those skills early in your life, and they will bode well later on. I am an adaptable person. And we have to be. My strengths are a willingness to adapt, to make changes, and to persevere—perhaps due to my genetics and necessity.

I enjoy learning more than anything, and I probably imbued that in my children by leaving books all over the house. My children are all engineers, but they also took liberal arts and science courses and are interested in things other than math and science.

I'm very fond of early American history. I think I could go to the East Coast and sit in seminars about the founding of our country and Jefferson and the founding fathers for days. YouTube can be an interesting learning experience, but caution is advised because to sift through the myriad videos in order to separate the excellent from the mediocre (or really worthless) eats up a lot of time. On the other hand, history programming on CSPAN over the weekends offers me unlimited access to great programs.

My daughter, Linda, and I had started doing some genealogy research. As I love history, it gave me something to bite into. I found out I'm 20 percent Jewish, as well as Irish and Italian, and have a newly discovered great-grandmother whose lineage starts in seventeenth-century Virginia. We were hoping our research may discover information that would lead to our family becoming involved with DAR and SAR—Daughters and Sons of the American Revolution. Along the way, I seem to have developed enough interests to keep me busy.

Linda passed away two years ago. I have a picture of her right here, and I look at her every day. I can talk about her a little bit now without crying or getting in a terribly morose state. It is unreal to me that she is gone. She was my only daughter; I have the three boys and daughters-in-law and their children—nine grandchildren altogether and a two-year-old great-grandson. I have started writing Linda's biography. It's very, very rough, but I'm determined to publish a little book of Linda's life. Right now it is handwritten, but I'm in the process of transferring it to a Word document, which I am trying to learn how to do.

I retired from Moraine Community College in 1999 and went to California. I enjoyed living in Monterey for two years. My mother's sister, Aunt Irene, was my closest connection to my mother, who died when I was four. The visit provided closure for me, perhaps having felt abandoned as a child.

Following my aunt's death and 9/11, I returned to Illinois and purchased a two-story residence listed as a colonial cottage. I bought the house for the garden, because I love to garden, and for the screen porch that went across the back. My best friend in high school had a house with a screen porch. Her family epitomized what I thought a family should be, and with the screen porch, I thought I was in heaven. When I saw this house with the screen porch, I knew I had to have it. Well, it has two floors, and seventeen years later, I'm paying the price for those stairs.

The last six months, it has been on my mind to downsize. I enjoy being on my screen porch, but there are things I can't do. I don't do the gardening anymore, although I still enjoy looking at the garden and seeing things grow. Now I want to move to a condo in a senior community, where I will have a good park district to take tai chi, and a great library I can walk to. Early on, I learned to creatively visualize my path forward, which has also been a very helpful tool. I know I need quiet time to rest, but I also need to reach out to friends individually and in groups.

In terms of aging, I don't deny my age. I am what I am. I can't do what I can't do. I feel the need to get out of the gloomy spells that do come, and I have people to live for. I lost Linda, who was not only my daughter but also my best friend. With one of my sons, I have something similar. We start talking about something and end up talking about the pyramids of Egypt and black holes.

One thing I became aware of as I approached eighty: Time now seems shorter. I have only so much time during the day when I feel mentally and physically able to participate—to go out for walks or go shopping or meet friends for lunch or go to my book club. In the afternoon, I come home from whatever I was doing, and I need quiet time. I need to sit back and regroup. That's the only time I can find to read, and I read a lot on my iPad. Thank God for that, because the libraries are all closed (due to COVID-19), and I can download books.

I know that older adults could benefit from simple procedures, such as downloading free books from their libraries. It has become a necessity for me. At night, I may wake up because my brain decides it needs to review all of my life's good and bad snapshots. I open my iPad and just start reading. I need to see the words, and then they fill the spaces where the difficulties of life insist on making themselves known.

I understand loneliness. I've had that, but it's in the past. I see my friends in book club and other activities, some of whom are my age and starting to lose spouses. I've already experienced and adjusted to being alone. I've been an independent person for so long that being alone doesn't bother me.

Something I realize as I'm getting older is the importance of friends. I never had a lot of girlfriends when I was young. I think it's critically important, especially as we are growing older. We have our children, yes, but we need our girlfriends for the gloomy spells that do come.

I'm losing height; I'm losing bone mass due to some osteopenia. Those are things I don't like; I rail against them. Then, I adapt. When I was about sixty-four, I started having surgeries. I've had both my knees and both hips replaced and two back surgeries. Last October, I had a heart attack—an emergency situation—so I have five stents now. Then, I signed up for ADT, a medical on-the-go alert service. It alleviates fear.

When I had the heart attack, luckily, I had ADT; I pushed the button, and the EMTs came. Another part of who I am is that I take care of what I need to.

Loneliness is dangerous. We need to reach out. We need to keep our friends and help others. I have always enjoyed talking with people, encouraging their potential as much as possible. Currently, I belong to a group of people who knit shawls for the sick. Being part of a group helps me to be much stronger than I know I would be alone.

Alan Ranford and Billie Teneau
Love in the Time of the Pandemic

Alan

Alan Ranford grew up in England during World War II. After he graduated from grammar school, he spent five years doing an apprenticeship with an engineering company and another six years at the local technical school, working toward a degree in engineering. He held jobs as a draftsman and an engineer in England, Canada, and the United States. His last job brought him to St Louis, Missouri, where he worked until he retired at seventy. Alan is now ninety-four.

We lived above the business in a small flat. When I was thirteen, the war started. We had some pretty lean years during the war, but we survived. I had no brothers or sisters; there wasn't room for more than one child in the flat. I was a very sickly child, and it wasn't until some remedies came along that my asthma was quelled somewhat. Inhalers came on the market when I was in my twenties.

After I earned my degree, I left my company and joined a radar research group as a draftsman. I took a trip to Switzerland with my parents, and it was there that I met my wife. We lived and worked in London for two years. We decided we weren't making enough money in England to have the life we wanted. The prospects didn't look good, so we emigrated to Canada and ended up in Toronto, where we lived for five-and-a-half years and enjoyed it very much.

After about a year in Toronto, we took a ten-thousand-mile tour around the States. During the trip, my wife had a tubal pregnancy. We barely saved her when we got back home, and after that she couldn't have children. So, we had to adopt. Fortunately, we had a very good adoption agency in Toronto, and we adopted a little girl. Then, we wanted a second child. We weren't due for one, but the agency went out of its way for us and found us a little boy.

I was working for a company that made instruments for high-speed interceptor aircraft. It was very successful, but the order was canceled. The only jobs available were in the States, so we moved to Grand Rapids, Michigan.

Eventually, the company I was working for in Grand Rapids began laying off people. While we were there, we had built our dream house on the bank of a river, and my wife had taken a four-year course in interior design. We moved to St. Louis, where I had a good job with a company that made disposable medical products. I worked there until I was seventy, while my wife carried on with her interior-design work.

I was a swimmer, and both of the houses I lived in had pools. The first house I had in St. Louis had a diving board. I made sure my children could swim, and I have three granddaughters who are all taking swimming lessons and swim extremely well. My children both lived in St. Louis. My son had a demanding job in the Aleutian Islands. He died at fifty-four with heart problems. My daughter was still working until COVID-19 happened. She was laid off, but she was at retirement age anyway. My wife died after our fiftieth anniversary.

When I met Billie, we fell for each other very quickly and have lived together for thirteen years. We had one date. We went to the art museum to see the Napoleon exhibit. Then Billie went to South Africa on a bike trip, which held things up for a little. She had a very nice house, so we decided to live there. We never saw the point of getting married. The secret of staying happy and coping with all the things that happen in life is having good partners.

Regarding race relations, and what is happening currently, older people are set in their thinking and haven't changed their views. The young people are thinking correctly. I am happy to see young white persons working with young Black persons in forming demonstrations and taking action. The Ethical Society has a Black Lives Matter demonstration periodically on Sundays (when we were having Sunday sessions). I guess time will tell what works, but if you speak to any Black person, he will tell you that, when he drives somewhere, he is almost surely going to get stopped. It's called driving while Black.

Billie

Billi Teneau grew up in small towns in Missouri until she was sixteen. She spent her senior year in Steel, another small town in the bootheel of Missouri. After graduation, she moved to St. Louis with her high school boyfriend, and they were married at eighteen. Her husband was drafted and lost part of his leg during WWII. After he recuperated, they both went to Washington University for one year. They were always interested in race relations. Billie became an important member of the Committee of Racial Equality (CORE), *planning and coordinating demonstrations at restaurant counters and working to pass legislation that made it illegal to deny service to any Black person in public accommodations. She was also an avid biker who traveled to several countries on biking trips.*

◆　◆　◆

Our home became the office for CORE, because as a stay-at-home mother with two children, I was there all the time. In addition to answering the telephone, I ran the office and wrote a newsletter. I helped to organize our frequent demonstrations, where we sat at restaurant counters on Saturday mornings for four or five hours at a time. We would sit in every other seat. This gave customers an opportunity to sit in the vacant seats, which they did. They asked questions, and we talked to them and invited them to share their concerns. Many people came over to our way of thinking. I also reported on the progress of our Saturday mornings in our newsletter.

At the same time, we were also dealing with organizations in St. Louis and getting them to submit information on the issues they were dealing with. In 1961, we got a bill passed in the St. Louis Board of Aldermen making it illegal to deny service to any Black person in public accommodations—primarily restaurants, but also theaters.

My husband and I divorced. My aim at that time was to go back to college and finish my degree, so that's what I did. I needed an inexpensive place to live and found that I qualified for living in the Pruitt Igoe housing project. My two children and I lived there for two-and-a-half years until I finished my degree. Then, we moved out to the county, and I got the first job I applied for as a teacher in Ferguson, Missouri, at the high school level in speech, drama, and English. I retired after thirty years but then taught for five more years in the city of St. Louis.

I had remarried, and my second husband died after I retired. I missed him very much, but there was nothing to do except keep going, so I did. Then, I met Alan at a memorial for our deceased spouses, where each of us was reduced to tears, and that was the beginning. Our first date was at the Art Museum. Things have gone very well now for about thirteen years. I just had my ninety-fifth birthday.

I go to physical therapy to make my legs a little more reliable because I still hope to do a little more riding on my bicycle. I was extremely involved in biking for several years. I had gone to the Netherlands twice; then, France; and most recently to South Africa. Alan and I both led some bike rides. It took two of us because I couldn't watch the end of a line of bikers, so I rode in the front of the line, and he rode in the back. If there were any real problems, it was up to him to handle them. We did that successfully the year before last and enjoyed it very much. I doubt we will lead rides again, but we will get around to doing some riding.

Aging—well, you can't stop it, but you can slow it down with a positive attitude and keeping a close watch on your own health. When you age, you find that the doctors are not calling you in as often. So, it takes some aggressiveness on the part of older people to be sure that you're getting the best healthcare.

Alan has been in better health than I have been. About two years ago I had a TIA—a small stroke—that kind of took me out of my biking action for a while. Then, I had the misfortune of falling due to a poorly designed parking lot. I tripped over the barrier that stops cars from going too far into the parking space. Since I was carrying some things in my left hand, I couldn't see well. The result was that I tripped and went down on my chin and my right arm. I broke my arm, and it took six months for that to heal. I fell on my chin. During my recovery, I spent entirely too much time sitting, and I needed very much to exercise and get mobile again. I am now taking PT to strengthen my legs to ride my bicycle.

My children are now at the age of contemplating retirement. I have three grandchildren and four great-grandchildren. They don't live close by, and for that I'm sorry. But that's the way it's worked out. My son lives in Georgia; my daughter lives in Washington, DC and has become an excellent online teacher of medical coding. She has written several books. Every time there's a change in coding, and they are frequent, she writes another book and has no trouble selling them.

My son was a manager of several kinds of stores and is retired. He is now seventy-two and has gone back to work because they needed somebody, but I think he was getting bored at home. He has carried on the tradition of working in race relations, but he's pretty sensible about it and is now at the age where he says it's time for the younger people to take over.

The secret of staying happy, as Alan said, is having good partners. But I would also add pursuing your own interests. When I was teaching drama, I directed many plays for my students that were open to the community. I also acted in community theater productions. My advice is, if you start doing something in your life, don't just drop it as you get older. Go forward, and keep doing it in some form or another.

As far as race relations in recent years, I found out there were teachers who were referring students to me as a reference on race relations and what approach we took. Our approach was not universal, but it was certainly known even then. It was entirely peaceful, but we were stubborn. We had demonstrations for hours every Saturday and marched in order to make our point. But at any of our demonstrations, if it looked like there might be some violence, or just plain old problems, we would leave the scene and come back another time. In terms of what's going on now, I do think the tide is turning.

II. GOING SOLO

Is it time to stop living on your own?

MOST LIKELY, if it's time to stop living on your own, your adult children will point this out to you before you realize it yourself. They may cite examples in which your behavior or appearance has changed—gently at first, but more bluntly as time goes on. Few subjects are more likely to stir up your emotions than this one. None of us wants to hear all the ways we could be a danger to ourselves if we are left alone. We might fall or forget to take our pills or skip meals or any of a dozen other ways we could be putting ourselves at risk.

Wasn't it only yesterday that you felt in charge of your life? Then overnight, you seem to need help doing all the things you've always done for yourself. Your family members have become detectives, pointing out that your clothes suddenly seem too big for you. Perhaps you have lost weight without even being aware of it? Has your appetite or interest in food decreased? Are you skipping meals? And on and on.

They notice everything. Have you stopped shaving or putting on makeup every day, breaking years of habits? Do you have a spot on your shirt because your laundry skills are slipping? Is unopened mail sitting in a pile on the table? Are you forgetting to pay bills? Are your breakfast dishes still in the sink? The list is endless, not to mention irritating. What has changed? Have you relaxed your standards, or are your children making mountains out of mole hills?

31

Who decides the time has come to reconsider your living arrangements—you or your family? Ideally, this is a team effort. Your role is to face the situation with an open mind and keep your emotions in check. Your children's role is to ask themselves what is really important and what isn't. And then, of course, delivery counts. What matters is not so much *what* they say as *how* they say it that can be hurtful. After all, you are still the parent and aren't quite ready to abandon that role.

Where to Find Help
There comes a time when this subject must be broached, despite your best efforts to avoid it. Even if you're managing quite well at the moment, there is no way to know what the future holds. How to handle life's inevitable changes isn't easy at best, so the words you and your children choose to talk about this really do matter.

Let's start with the hard part first—when you realize you really can't do all the things you used to be able to do and you need some help. What kind of help and how much of it you need ranges from having someone come in to clean once a week to downsizing your belongings and moving into a retirement home. In between those two extremes are a great many options; chances are you are not even aware of some of them. For example, there are not-for-profit organizations and government agencies that are devoted to providing help to senior citizens. Here are a few examples of national resources:

Elder Helpers (www.elderhelpers.org)
Elder Helpers is a free, user-friendly, Web-based service in which volunteers offer their services to help older people. The Elder Helpers program strives to safely and conveniently connect dedicated volunteers with elders in their local communities. The program is a tax-exempt nonprofit established in the United States in 2008.

Area Agencies on Aging & Services (www.health.mo.gov/seniors/aaa)
The federal Older Americans Act (OAA) requires all states to establish Area Agencies on Aging (AAA). Each area agency develops and implements programs for older persons at the local level. These include legal services; nutrition, including home-delivered meals; in-home services, such as chores, personal or respite care; disease prevention and health promotion; transportation assistance; and advocacy. AAAs are also expected to provide any combination of the following services: friendly visits, assistance with health education, minor home repair, and recreation.

National Council on Aging (NCOA) (www.ncoa.org)
NCOA offers more than 2,500 benefit programs nationwide for medication, healthcare, income assistance, food and nutrition, housing and utilities, tax relief, veterans, employment, economic security, healthy living, public policy, blogs and news, getting involved, and resources. Under each of these categories are numerous programs ranging from preventing falls and managing the aging process to income assistance.

Even more sources of support for seniors are available, but all you need in this age of the Internet are a few good search engines to help you find them. When we think of search engines, in addition to Google, Bing, Yahoo, Ask.com, AOL.com, Baidu, Wolframalpha, DuckDuckGo, Internet Archive, and Yandex.ru make up the ten most popular search engines in the world (as of 2019). For variety's sake, it might be fun to try out some of the less familiar ones.

If all of those choices make your head spin, there are some more obvious solutions you have probably already considered. When you realize that your health is failing or grocery shopping and cooking have become a chore, it's obvious you could use some help. You may find it through the national agencies listed above, such as the Area Agency on Aging in your state or more local organizations in your community.

Many of these services are provided at no cost, while others do charge a fee. If you have long-term health insurance that covers in-home care or can afford to hire someone on a part-time or full-time basis, those are excellent alternatives as well.

A long-term healthcare policy usually covers the cost of a retirement community that would allow you to move from independent living to assisted living to long-term care, depending on your needs. If you can afford such an arrangement without insurance, be aware that this will be one of your more expensive options.

Another possibility you should think through carefully before you decide to give it a try is moving in with your adult children. For some older people this works very well, but be aware of a number of caveats. If your relationship with your children has always been a bit fraught, suddenly sharing their home is unlikely to improve it. Ask yourself these questions: Do your children have enough room for an additional person (or two, if you are married), especially one who might require extra care? Would you have your own room, and would it provide both privacy and the personal touches that would make it feel like home? Have you clarified the house rules in advance? Will you feel like a burden, even if your children assure you that is not the case?

This subject could fill a book of its own, and if it is something you are seriously considering, take the time to do a little research. Every decision you make regarding how and where you will live the rest of your life is hugely important, but few are as potentially emotional as reversing the natural order of things by moving back in with your adult children.

The Way We Were

One more thought on this subject: Once upon a time, not so many years ago, several family members lived under the same roof, and these multigenerational arrangements were neither unusual nor traumatic. Everyone provided support when it was needed, and children developed close relationships with their grandparents and other older relatives. In many ways, these arrangements were healthy and natural—more natural, in fact, than families spread out across the country in our present mobile society. Having spent several years living with my grandmother, I can't help feeling that something has been lost in our newly evolved nuclear families.

Because people are living longer, six distinct generations make up the US population today. Over time, each of these generations has been nicknamed based on the behavior of its young people and historical events that have molded their personalities. Currently, the largest of these groups is the Baby Boomers, born between 1946 and 1964, many of whom have already joined the ranks of retirees. Numerous inventions we take for granted these days were created to meet the needs of the Baby Boomers who will soon be asking the same question you are grappling with now: *Is it time to stop living alone?*

Any one of the solutions proposed earlier in this chapter might well serve their needs, but they don't quite fill the bill because most Baby Boomers don't want to live with their children or move to a retirement community. They want to stay exactly where they are, in their own homes. In other words, they want to "age in place." Aging in place describes how people are able to live wherever they choose, as long as they can do so safely, and have access to any support they might require as their needs change.

While the terminology may sound new, the concept of aging in place has been around since the seventies and is once again gaining popularity as more and more Baby Boomers enter their retirement years. Another related idea making a comeback is that of "universal design." According to the Disability Act of 2005, universal design describes the design of buildings, products, or environments that make them accessible by all people, regardless of their age, size, ability, or disability. Aging in place will become more feasible when universal design is incorporated into new structures in their early planning stages.

If universal design were a common practice today, more adults would find it easier to remain in their homes for longer periods of time. But until such time as universal design is considered a routine element in building homes, people who want to stay put are going to have to be creative in bringing their living spaces up to speed.

If You Really Want to Stay Home

You probably love where you live—which may be anywhere from a mobile home to a mansion—and hope to stay there for the rest of your life. Right this minute, everything about it works well for your lifestyle. You can't imagine changing a thing, and yet deep down, you know that as the years add up, you will need to make a few adjustments here and there. Perhaps you live in a two-story house with the bedrooms upstairs. While you can climb those stairs with ease right now, that might not always be the case. Walking around your house poses no problem now, but what if you had to use a walker for a while? Would it get stuck in your doorways and bump into furniture in an overcrowded room?

You have probably never have thought about these potential problems, but they are only two on a long list of issues you will have to address eventually. Your comfortable house may be full of hidden booby-traps. Nearly half of all injuries suffered by older people occur at home, especially falling, and sometimes your biggest problem isn't poor balance as much as it is vanity. If you have a cane or walker, for goodness sake, use it! Ask yourself which is worse: using an assistive device to walk or landing on your rear end in a public place? One of the worst parts about falling, besides the risk of serious injury, isn't feeling embarrassed; it is feeling helpless.

All it takes is one fall to destroy our confidence in our own stability. After falling once, I became more careful about how and where I was walking. Sometimes I have found it easier not to walk at all, which then puts me at risk of weakening my legs. Inactivity may keep me from falling, but it has consequences of its own. The more you move, the stronger your muscles become; the stronger your muscles, the less likely you are to fall.

Slipping on a wet floor in a grocery store or tripping over a curb as you cross the street is not that unusual for older people, but surprisingly, they don't happen as often as falling in your own home. As you walk through your house, be on the lookout for potential dangers. The number one risk factor is clutter— items left on the floor, piles of magazines, books, toys (if you have grandchildren), partially finished mending, arts and crafts projects, throw rugs, wet towels in the bathroom, and clothes you meant to hang up but never got around to doing it. Maybe that's why there are so many books on the market on clearing your clutter with everything from Feng Shui to Swedish death cleaning.

Leaving things lying around or forgetting to pick them up is a symptom of flitting from one task to another without even realizing you're doing it. This can be even more dangerous when those tasks involve leaving a pot cooking on the stove or the water running in the sink. While it's not likely that these are symptoms of dementia, they are a sign that your mind is wandering. Lack of concentration can occur at any age but is particularly hazardous to the elderly, and the reasons often have more to do with the state of your health than the state of your memory.

If you set the timer on your stove but don't hear it go off, the problem may be your hearing. If the food in your pantry or refrigerator is far past its sell-by date, or you have misread a prescription label, it may be time to have your eyes checked. If you find yourself skipping appointments or losing track of time, it could be because of short-term memory loss or, even more likely, lack of organization. The older I get, the more I realize how important it is to make lists and keep my calendar up to date. We are living in an era of information overload—when we take in more details than we are able to process. This phrase is more apropos today than when it was first introduced by futurist Alvin Toffler in his groundbreaking book, *Future Shock*, published in 1970. And there was far less information to sort through fifty years ago.

Before you panic about your lack of organization, take an honest inventory of your health. If you suspect you don't see or hear as well as you used to, or you find yourself searching for words or names that have slipped your mind, don't deny your own instincts. On the other hand, you may be relieved to find the problem isn't as serious as you anticipated. Whatever the issue may be, once you know what you're dealing with, it makes no sense to deny the obvious. If you need cataract surgery or hearing aids or even a total knee replacement, delaying the inevitable will not improve your comfort level and, in a worst-case scenario, may make it difficult for you to remain in your home.

Aging in place does not mean sitting in your favorite chair and hoping for the best. You have a significant role to play in staying as healthy and alert as possible for as long as possible. It may not be feasible to take care of yourself, your house, and your spouse, if you have one, without help. But help is available in many forms, which brings us right back to the beginning of this chapter.

While it's true that our concentration often slips with the passage of time, there is a way to deal with that problem. Like so many ideas that seem brand new, this one is actually ancient. It is called "mindfulness." It is more than 2,500 years old and is practiced all over the world. According to the American Psychological Association (APA), mindfulness is "a moment-to-moment awareness of one's experience without judgment." Jon Kabat Zinn, who is known worldwide for his work on mindfulness-based stress reduction (MBSR), advises that we focus our attention "right here, right now"—again, without judging. In an age of social media, where opinions, likes, and judgment are ubiquitous, it's easy to see how this could come as a relief.

Besides freeing us from the unsolicited opinions of everyone who has one to share, mindfulness has another practical use: It keeps your attention from wandering off in all directions. Decades ago, Ram Das, a student of Eastern religions, wrote a book called *Be Here Now*, and I have never found a better definition of mindfulness. It simply means that wherever you are, be fully present. Whatever you are doing, pay attention. Whatever is going on around you, be aware of what is happening.

If you form the habit of living mindfully, you are less likely to lose track of what you're doing. You won't leave the stove on or the water running, lose track of your appointments, or trip on clutter you forgot to pick up off the floor. You will, as Ram Das urged in the simplest of words, *Be Here Now*. If *here* is home, what better place is there to be?

Here's What You Can Do to Eliminate Risks

How do you know when it's time to face the need for help, either in your own home or in an assisted living facility? The biggest clue is when you find yourself falling. Falling is frightening, as well as an indication that your mobility is becoming more limited. But before you pack up your house and prepare to move, there are number of things you can do to ameliorate this potential problem. First, admit that it is happening. You may be able to keep this a secret from friends and family, but you can't fool yourself. Second, decide what you going to do about it. Short of rehabbing your whole house, there are number of steps you can take that are much more practical, not to mention less expensive.

Pick up a laundry basket, and take a walk around your house. What you are looking for is every possible item that could trip you up when you're not paying attention. The most obvious culprits are anything on the floor, from magazines and newspapers to clothes you've just dropped and forgotten about. If you have grandchildren, there may be toys, some as hard to see as Legos and puzzle pieces. Just scoop everything off the floor. That means *everything*. You can always empty the laundry basket later.

Whenever you're up to another walk through, check out your furniture. Anything that sticks out or is sitting in the middle of a room, such as chair or couch legs, footboards on beds, benches, footstools, small ladders, plants, and especially electrical cords, all pose potential threats. If you have tripped on something in the past, try to see how you can change its position in the room or move it someplace else.

The kitchen is another danger spot. If it's cluttered with furniture that doesn't really need to be there, move it to another room, your storage area, or get rid of it altogether. Be sure your electrical cords are not hanging over the counter or all tangled up. Besides smoothing them out and tucking them out of sight, you might want to unplug them at night when you're no longer using the kitchen.

The throw rug in your bathroom poses another problem. To keep from slipping on the floor, buy nonslip bathroom rugs to be sure they don't move. You should have nonslip pads or strips in your bathtub or shower and grab bars on the walls to keep you steady. At a certain point, getting in and out of the bathtub becomes difficult, but there are tubs with doors that allow you to just step right in and even sit down. If you have a walk-in shower, which is a good alternative to a bathtub, be sure your shower floor is level with no trim you could possibly trip over.

If you have stairs in your home, you should have banisters on both sides of the staircase so you can hold on whether you're walking up or down the stairs. If the stairs are wood, have strips installed on each step to keep you from slipping.

The point of all of this is that you must begin to look at your home with new eyes so that you can identify any potential hazard that has probably never occurred to you before. If all of these suggestions sound a little over-the-top, believe me, you will be grateful for the time you spent eliminating the harmless-looking obstacles that could land you on the floor. Every fall you don't have extends not only your life but the *quality* of your life as well.

Ellen Brasunas
Aging in Place

Ellen Brasunas is ninety-five. She has lived in the same home for more than fifty years, and she plans to remain there. She has looked at other options and decided to age in place, with a little help from Home Instead, an agency that makes it possible for the elderly to remain in their homes. Ellen has been a nurse and a counselor for most of her life. She lost her husband and soulmate in 2000, but being a life-long meditator has helped her cope with the loss. [Ellen passed away at ninety-six, five months after this interview.]

◆　◆　◆

I was a nurse, an RN, and a psychiatric nurse. I was in nursing for a long time, and then I went back and got my master's in counseling. I was in private practice for thirty-eight years. Toward the end, I cut my client load down, and then I just stopped. I was doing mostly individuals, but sometimes I would see couples for marriage counseling.

I've been meditating for over thirty years. I don't know that it has directly influenced my counseling, but meditation has helped me handle stress, which in turn, I guess, helped my clients. I didn't use meditation in counseling; I didn't teach meditation unless somebody wanted to learn. Because it affected me, I guess it did affect the way I interacted with them.

I've lived in my house for fifty-two years. As I got older, I did look at other options but ultimately decided to stay here. I went to quite a few places, and both of my daughters said I could come and stay with them. But I just love my home. I love my independence. I love that I can eat what I want when I want. Last night, I made a stew with rice and ate at 9:30pm.

When I was deciding what to do, I looked at assisted-living facilities. I wanted to be close to where most of my friends are and the Ethical Society, which I had belonged to for many years. Every place I looked at was quite far away from where I had lived all these years.

My son, Jim, lives nearby. He doesn't come over too much now because of the coronavirus pandemic. But you know, if anything goes wrong with the house, he supervises getting it taken care of. I've put him in charge of my money, although he doesn't handle all of it. We talk about my income and whatever I need around the house.

My house has two stories. Attached to the living room is a room where I used to hold counseling sessions. I moved downstairs, and that's where my bedroom is now. The room looks out on the backyard. When people want to come to visit me, I put a chair out there in the back yard so they can look into my picture window. I'll be inside, and whoever comes to visit me will be outside. Then, we will both talk on our cell phones. But my niece came over the other day, and we sat outside—six feet apart—and we both wore masks.

I wake up in the morning because the women from Home Instead are here every day from nine to noon. I can't speak highly enough of them. I'm pretty sure Home Instead is a national franchise, because my daughter in Arizona is the one who told me about them. She went online, and she said "Mom, this sounds like a wonderful arrangement for you." It has worked out beautifully. They're very conscious of what I need, and they're very kind people. As I understand it, the man who runs this company is really a fine person.

Ellen's motto is *to learn, to love, and to serve.* It must be synchronicity that she wrote a poem called "Going Solo."

How many nights together in 60 years?
Nights of sleeping, spooning, touching, and loving.
Now, he's disappeared.

Where has he gone, my friend, companion, and lover?
I reach out to emptiness.
Every day, we had our morning routine.
He would shave while I would exercise, then coffee together.
Indoors or out, a walk to the church and around "the hook"
We'd kiss under the pine tree and laugh if one of us would forget.
What joy and contentment we shared!
Today, with some tears (not too many), I have thought—
We really had it made!
Going Solo is a new adventure for me.
I'll make it with a little help from my friends and family.
I'm resilient.

Robin Garnett
Choosing Assisted Living

Robin Garnett is an LPN with more than twenty years' experience working with older adults in skilled nursing, memory care, assisted living, and post-acute care. Robin has been with Lutheran Senior Services for twelve years and has worked as a charge nurse, household coordinator, health-service counselor, and clinical liaison. As director of health services, she oversees the care of residents in assisted living and assisted-living memory care.

◆ ◆ ◆

One of the big advantages of living in an assisted-living community is the ability to maintain your independence while receiving the level of assistance you need to remain safe. This doesn't mean that someone oversees your every move or that you have a babysitter; you have the level of independence that is safe and comfortable for you. When you are at home, alone, there is a certain level of risk. If you have a fall or an injury, you may have to wait for an extended period before some-one is available to help. In assisted living, you have someone close by twenty-four hours a day. There is also someone who is well versed in healthcare and available to act as your advocate when you are working with physicians and during hospital stays, which can be a difficult time for anyone.

A really positive aspect of assisted living is the socialization. Often, as we age, our world actually grows smaller. Our friends are aging as well, and we may not be as physically able to get together as we used to. Driving after dark, or at all, becomes difficult, and hearing loss can make staying in touch via telephone difficult. Coming to a community gives you the opportunity to make new friends or connect with old ones from earlier in life. That happens more often than you'd think!

Of course, nothing is perfect, and there can be some things that feel challenging when you make the move to assisted living. It can be difficult to admit the need for assistance for those who have been independent all their lives. Asking for help, no matter how little, can be hard to do. It's also true that most of us aren't usually the best judge of what we need. Things change so slowly that we may not notice how difficult a task has become until we're relieved of that task, such as mowing the lawn. This can seem like a loss of independence.

Moving into a community means there will be less space for "stuff." Often, as our world becomes smaller socially, we tend to collect physical things to fill that hole. We're also working with the reality of a lifetime of things, both ours and our children's and perhaps our grandchildren's. Fortunately, there are companies that are available to assist with declut-tering and downsizing. These companies will come into your home, help you choose what you want or need to bring with you and what to let go of. Letting go can entail donating, having family members (finally) come collect their things, selling items, or just tossing whatever is of no further value. These companies will also help you move and get settled in your new space. Some companies, such as Lutheran Senior Services (LSS), even offer this service at no charge for new moves.

A good candidate for assisted living is someone who doesn't wait too long to enjoy the benefits this living arrangement has to offer. The ability to maintain your independence with oversight is a significant benefit. But if you wait until you need more help than an assisted- living level of care can provide, you will miss out on these benefits.

Assisted living offers the chance to be social with others. It is community living after all, and you are sharing space. It's a good idea to think about how you interact with others before making the decision to move. If you treasure solitude over socializing, of if you truly "don't play well with others," assisted living may not be right for you. But, in my experience, those are pretty rare situations.

I can't stress enough the importance of gathering information and doing your research. Find out what assisted living is and is not. Being realistic about your needs and capabilities is very important when you are considering making this transition. Making a list of what's important to you can help you know what to look for in a community. For example, if keeping your dog with you is at the top of your list, you would know not to look at communities that don't allow pets.

Take tours of communities and request information. Ask lots of questions, take notes, and focus on your list of things that really matter. Finally, talk with your family about your possible move. Let them know what you are considering and why, discuss their ideas, and listen to what they have to say. But, remember, you are the one who will make the decision.

One of the positive aspects of being in a community is that the ability to face a crisis, such as COVID-19, is built in. We have been able to keep our residents safe by the early intervention of safety measures. By living in a community, our residents don't have to worry about trips to the grocery store, medication management and delivery, or remaining healthy and safe while trying to handle daily tasks. Our staff is monitored and utilizes safety measures to handle these tasks for our residents. By being in a community, you will have the full power of dedicated healthcare professionals with years of experience making decisions that will keep you as safe as possible.

Dealing with this unprecedented pandemic has been a challenge for sure. We did have to honor the shelter-in-place order that was announced earlier this year by having residents stay in their apartments for a time. We all worked very hard to retain the connection and socialization that is such an important part of the life of a community.

Our activity department has been very creative in keeping people entertained and connected. Examples are Skype calls with residents and their families, hallway bingo and happy hours, strolling strings, exercise classes shown on TV, and meal delivery to apartments. Some residents said they felt like they saw people even more often during this time, since staff was in the apartments so often, checking in, delivering medication, and visiting!

As the older adult, you are the person who makes the final decision. Adult children or family members have their opinions and ideas, but the decision is always yours, and we support that.

Objections usually come from a place of fear or uncertainty. The best we can do is answer the questions, explain how things work as carefully as we can, share information and be transparent, and try to make the idea of moving more comfortable. Frequent objections are the denial of the need to move, reluctance to give up the family home, and attachment to a lifetime of mementos and keepsakes. In my experience, as in most uncertain situations in life, it's the anticipation and fear of the unknown that is the scary part. Once the decision is made and the move is completed, the results are very positive.

At Lutheran Senior Services, we offer a program called Benevolent Care, in which we make a commitment to the people who choose to move in with us. Residents make a promise to use their resources to provide for their care for as long as they can. We make a commitment to those people to care for them for the remainder of their lives regardless of continued financial ability. There are communities that do not have the ability to accept Medicaid and do not have the programs we have. These communities would require residents to find alternate places to live when their financial resources are exhausted.

Activities in assisted living are as varied as the residents who live with us. We offer group activities, of course, but there are also so many opportunities for residents to be active on their own or in small groups. We have residents who play bridge weekly, paint, knit, watch TV and movies, and do puzzles together. Some residents enjoy reading, and others are more social and want to be a part of all the group outings. We have exercise classes, one-on-one visits with chaplains and activity staff, musical groups, drumming, chime choir, and crafts. When we're not dealing with a pandemic, we go on shopping trips, eat in restaurants, visit museums, and see plays and movies.

Making the choice to move to assisted living can seem daunting, but if you take your time, gather the information, ask the right questions, and choose the right community, it can be the best move you've ever made. You are actually making the decision to maintain your independence, because, now you will receive the assistance you need to do all the things you haven't been able to do for some time.

III. GETTING SERIOUS ABOUT SAFETY

What does it take to accident-proof your surroundings?

I DON'T KNOW OF TOO MANY OLDER PEOPLE who go quietly into the night without putting up one hell of a fight. I surely am not one of them. No matter when anyone suggests some device that is obviously in my best interest, I don't think I need it. I don't need a cane; I don't need tennis shoes that tie instead of slip on; and I certainly don't need one of those emergency alert medallions (the "help-me-I've fallen-and-I-can't-get-up" buttons) to wear around my neck. They are unattractive and all-too-obvious announcements of my encroaching frailty. I fought having one every inch of the way until I finally caved in to pressure and said okay. Even then, I refused to wear anything around my neck. I consented to the bracelet, which, unless you looked closely, resembled a Fitbit or an Apple watch. The device came in two colors—black and white—was waterproof and nearly indestructible, and had the annoying trait of calling me if one of my daughters couldn't find me.

After a few months, I forgot the bracelet was even on my wrist. Then, one morning, I remembered. I awoke at 3:30 AM unable to breathe. I guess I didn't assess the situation very quickly because I walked around for an hour trying to catch my breath and figure out what to do. Only then did I think to push the button on my bracelet. The bracelet asked me what the problem was, and I said, "I'm having trouble breathing."

Five minutes later the EMTs arrived (lots of them), along with oxygen and a stretcher, and I was whisked away in an ambulance to the nearest hospital.

That was my first ambulance ride, and I wish I could remember it or being in the emergency room. By that time—about 5 AM—my daughter had arrived and kindly spared me the I-told-you-so lecture. The diagnosis was pneumonia, the hospital stay was four days, and I was sent home with oxygen. As medical experiences go, this one was pretty positive. I even wrote a letter to the CEO, singing the nursing staff's praises. The point of this story isn't the speed and efficiency of the EMTs, the TLC of the medical staff, or even that the CEO answered my letter, but rather that little button on my wrist, which probably saved my life.

I've seen that commercial a hundred times at least but never felt it had any connection to me. It wasn't until I had fallen a few times that I realized just how vulnerable I was. No matter how old people are, they are at risk of falling. Anyone can slip on ice, miss a step walking down the stairs, trip over an unseen wire, or simply lose her balance. And that's just outside. Indoors, there are hidden hazards everywhere you look or, more accurately, where you don't look. Few of us walk around our homes looking at the floors, which is a good reason for removing items that can trip you up before they do.

I learned this the hard way, which is the way most of us learn life's lessons. I tripped over a big, fat pillow and hit the floor hard. The room looked like a crime scene with blood everywhere. I looked even worse. I had a gash down the side of my face and several cuts and bruises in other places, all of which were bleeding profusely. The next day, I had a huge, dark purple and pink black-eye, and my eye had swollen shut. I was covered in bandages and spent a week putting ice packs on my eye to reduce the swelling; the intense purple patch took much longer to fade.

What did I learn? Lesson number one: If you're supposed to be using a walker, by all means, use it. It is of little use if it's in another room or out in the car, where mine happened to be. Lesson number two: If you know you're going to get up during the night, make sure the area around your bed is clear. It doesn't matter if the offending obstacle is a big stuffed pillow or a small stuffed animal. They are equally dangerous.

The World Then and Now

At the risk of sounding overly dramatic, we live in dangerous times. I tend to forget that because I was raised in the fifties, a pretty benign decade when the word *fear* wasn't in our vocabulary. We played outside unsupervised for hours, we walked to school, and we lived without security systems. Life wasn't exactly like an episode from *Father Knows Best*, but it was close.

We took safety for granted back then, which is something most of us don't do today. And we are wise to take such matters seriously. "The most essential human need—beyond the necessity for air, water, and food—is to be safe. It is even more essential to life than to be loved." That is the first paragraph in the first chapter of *Think Safe, Be Safe: The Only Guide to Inner Peace and Outer Security* by Harold H. Bloomfield MD and Robert K. Cooper, PhD, both experts in the field of safety and security.

The national survey on fear of crime, *The Figgie Report*, indicates that "four out of five Americans are afraid of being assaulted, robbed, raped, or murdered. Being constantly afraid may kill you faster than violence itself." This is particularly relevant to older people, because an ongoing fear for personal safety can systematically destroy brain cells, which accelerates the aging of your mind. The author's philosophy is to become aware of potential dangers, make sensible plans for actions you can take, and then put an end to chronic worry about safety.

Don't Be Afraid—Be Prepared

Fear feeds on itself. Once fear takes hold, it doesn't let go easily, but you don't have to be a victim of all the things that *could* happen to you as you get older. For every potential danger you can think of, there are numerous preventive actions you can take to keep yourself safe. While some of them will require outside assistance, you can do many things to protect yourself. Being proactive is a confidence builder, and it's hard to be confident and fearful at the same time.

Start with the big picture, because no one can tackle the many facets of safety all at once. Take a wide-angle view of the situation. Consider the following:

- Your home
- Stairs, floors, and carpeted areas
- Your kitchen
- Your car
- Intruders
- Falling
- Your personal safety and security
- An active mind and body
- Cyberspace
- Food poisoning
- Finances

That's a lot to think about, but awareness does not have to become paranoia. Information is power. The more you know about the risks involved, the better prepared you can be to deal with them. What follows is an exhaustive list of suggestions for each of the above safety issues. They may not all be relevant to your situation; they may not all be possible to implement; or they may be things you have already done. But the list is worth keeping for future reference.

Protect Yourself at Home
Your home is supposed to be your sanctuary—the place you feel safest— but the older you are, the less safe you may feel unless you take some necessary precautions. You can no longer take for granted the things you never thought about when you were younger, such as toys scattered

around the living room or clothes dropped on the floor instead of in the hamper. The sixth sense that kept you from tripping on items in the past may not be as sharp today. If you aren't aware of what is around you, your home can easily turn into an obstacle course.

- Take a room-by-room inventory of what is out of place, on the floor, making a mess, or posing a risk of tripping.
- Declutter your house one room at a time. If decluttering doesn't come naturally to you, you couldn't have picked a better time to try your hand at it. Amazon lists 2,000 books on decluttering, so you shouldn't have any trouble finding the help you need.
- Eliminate footstools, coffee tables, and anything with sharp edges you can trip over or bump into.
- Remove scatter rugs and carpets from stairs to prevent slipping.
- If you have stairs, clear everything off of them.
- Have at least one armchair that is easy to get in and out of.
- Check out your shoes to be sure they fit well and have non-slip soles. Velcro straps can be easier to tighten or loosen.
- Install better, brighter lighting to make sure you can see everything in the room.
- Check the location of light switches, and have them moved if they can't be easily reached by someone in a wheelchair.
- Get rid of defective or broken outdoor furniture.
- Don't leave toys, bicycles, or equipment in the driveway.

Protect Yourself on Stairs, Floors, and Carpeted Areas

Dropped clothes or forgotten toys left on the stairs become tripping and falling hazards. Aging eyes may not always be able to separate one step from the next, causing potential stumbles. After surgery or at a certain age, people may not be able to climb steps at all. Grabbing a loose hand-rail can be more dangerous than not having a handrail at all. Floors and carpeted areas are easy to ignore but can be the source of all kinds of potential hazards—things you look at every day but don't really see. To look where you're going and keep an eye on the floor at the same time can be difficult, which is the best reason to keep the floor uncluttered.

- Clear everything off the stairs.
- Install handrails on both sides of the stairs; tighten stair handrails both inside and outside the house.
- Consider a chairlift if climbing stairs becomes too difficult.
- Shovel snow and chip ice off stairs in the winter. Delegate this job to a younger family member, or hire a neighbor.
- Tuck away power strips and extension cords behind furniture to prevent tripping. Tape down any cords that can't be hidden.
- Stuff pillows in plush armchairs to make it easier to get up.

Protect Yourself in the Kitchen

Though you may not think about this, many hazards are hiding in your kitchen. Things you take for granted, such as your small appliances and cutlery. Of course, your stove and oven present their own kind of risks. Staying mindful of what you're doing is particularly important in this room.

- Turn off all stove burners when you leave the kitchen unless you are making something that has to simmer. If that's the case, set a timer in the kitchen and on your watch or smart phone.
- Don't leave anything cooking on the stove or in the oven when you leave the house.
- Be careful when you pour hot liquids from one container to another.
- If you have small children nearby, remind them frequently about the dangers of a hot stove.
- Be sure your countertops are easy to reach and large enough to work on. If you are in a wheelchair, have a contractor lower your countertops for ease of use.
- Keep sharp knives in drawers or special knife holders and away from the edge of counters. Sharpen them regularly, because dull knives are dangerous to use.

- Check your faucets to make sure they are easy to turn on and off. When you walk away from the sink, be sure they are off.
- If you spill something on the floor, clean it up immediately. Wet spots on the floor are a common cause of falls.
- Keep your cleaning supplies together in a safe place out of the reach of children. Do not mix two different cleaning supplies together. If you run out of one, replace it.
- If you have grandchildren who love to open cabinets, put ties on the handles to keep the doors closed.
- Don't place items you need on high shelves that require a bench or stepladder to reach. Avoid using a stepladder when you are alone. If possible, ask someone to hand you what you need.

Protect Yourself in Your Car

If you are still driving, there are several things you should be aware of, including your eyesight, reflexes, flexibility, and knowledge of the rules of the road. If you're honest with yourself, you know that some of these things have changed over the years. There are more cars on the road than ever, and driving has become a defensive sport no matter how old you are. That's all the more reason to take precautions as a driver.

- Research the rules and requirements for senior drivers from the Department of Motor Vehicles in your state.
- When you're in your car, keep the doors locked at all times. Don't leave your car windows wide open. Open them wide enough to give you adequate air but not enough to allow someone to reach into your car.
- Service your car regularly, at the times recommended by your car dealer or as soon as you become aware of some little tool lighting up on your dashboard.
- Drive on routes you've driven before and are familiar with. Use a GPS—either the one built into your car or on your cell phone.
- Always wear your seatbelt.

- If you have a purse or backpack, put it on the floor, not on the seat next to you. Keep your valuable items in your trunk.
- Avoid driving at night as soon as you find it difficult to do so. If you must drive at night, be sure to travel on well-lit streets. Whenever possible, don't drive alone.
- Park in a well-lit area, as close to an entrance as possible. Ask a police officer or security guard to accompany you back to your car when you leave a store at night.
- Don't keep personal information on your keychain.

Protect Yourself from Intruders

Few of us live in small towns where everyone knows everyone and no one locks their doors. Learn to protect yourself from unwanted guests, especially in urban environments. If you want to feel safe in your home, there are several steps you can take to assure your security.

- To make your home safer, consider a reputable security system, doors and windows with sturdy locks, good outside lighting, and even motion sensors.
- Display easily visible alarm-system signs in the front and back of your home and security-system decals on outside windows.
- Arrange for a free home-security inspection by contacting the crime prevention unit of your local police department. Most precincts will send an officer to your home to identify any doors, windows, or locks that need to be strengthened or secured.
- Install a wide-angle door viewer or peephole at each exterior door. If a stranger comes to your door, don't pretend you're not home. Check the peephole to verify the person's identity and reason for being there. If you are uncomfortable, call the police.
- When you are away, create the illusion that you are still at home. Use lamps that go on automatically at a certain time, and leave the TV on.
- Make your house numbers easy to read so that police can identify your home if they are called.

- Be sure your exterior doors are made of solid core wood or metal.
- Put window locks and security latches on sliding glass doors.
- Install a security-locking garage door (one that uses secure rolling code technology to prevent easy interception or opening remotely).
- Have your shrubs and bushes around the house trimmed to waist height.
- Limit the number of trees around your house's perimeter.
- Illuminate entrance areas and walkways using exterior floodlights with a motion-detector switch.
- Install a hidden security wall vault for storing valuables and important papers.
- Be sure your window shades or blinds cover the entire window.
- Put reliable smoke detectors in each zone of your home, and change the batteries on a regular basis.
- Make your bedroom into a safe room by installing a strong doorframe and solid core door with a deadbolt lock and a hard strike plate.

Protect Yourself from Falling

Falling is something we would rather not think about, let alone discuss. But the older we get, the more common and risky falling becomes. The Centers for Disease Control and Prevention reports that "more than one out of four older people falls each year, but less than half tell their doctor." What's more, falling once doubles your chances of falling again.

And that is only part of the picture. According to a World Health Organization (WHO) report, falls lead to 10-15 percent of all emergency-room visits. People over sixty-five account for more than 50 percent of injury-related hospitalizations due to conditions ranging from hip fractures to traumatic brain injuries. Older people's bones become brittle and can easily break in a fall. As frightening as those numbers are, even more so is that falls are responsible for 40 percent of all injury deaths.

Much less obvious are the effects of even the smallest fall on our self-confidence and sense of independence. If a fall happened once, it can happen again and often does. You might be tempted to keep repetitive falling a secret or even deny that you have fallen more than once or twice. Often, the only way our adult children know there is a problem is if they witness it happening. Those of us who have fallen more than once often become overcautious about going places. Repeated falls can cause once-confident elders to become timid and tentative in our movements. When a parent falls, our children tend to become overly vigilant in monitoring our safety. While they are trying to protect us from harm, we may misinterpret their concern as a threat to our independence, turning the situation into a Catch-22.

Since maintaining our independence is important to all of us as we grow older, we need to be proactive in reducing our risk of falling. This is not a responsibility we can leave to others. Most falls occur in the home, so your first step should be to do a risk assessment. Walk around your living space, and take a clear-eyed look at obvious and not-so-obvious obstacles.

Wet surfaces in the kitchen or bathroom can be very dangerous, and older people often lack the balance and reaction time needed to avoid a fall. Stepping out of a shower may seem a simple task, but an unsteady older person may slip and come crashing to the floor.

- Be sure bathmats have nonskid bottoms.
- Put nonslip mats in the bathtub and shower.
- Install grab bars inside the shower stall or just above the bathtub.
- Put in a shower seat to make showering safer and more comfortable.
- Replace the showerhead with a handheld one.

Protect Your Personal Safety and Security

Unexpected accidents are not the only events that merit your attention. Even if you live in what is considered a "safe neighborhood," that doesn't mean you could never be a victim of a crime. Whether you are at home or out shopping, walking down the street, entering or leaving your home, or driving, be as vigilant as possible.

- Wherever you are, be aware of your surroundings and people who are nearby.
- Don't go out at night by yourself. Ask a relative or friend to go with you. Make it a point to be around other people.
- If you take cabs or use Uber, Lyft, or other private-ride services, stay awake and alert, and avoid personal conversations with the driver.
- Never leave your purse unattended, such as in a grocery cart, while you shop. If you do use a purse, get one that straps across your body or use a fanny pack.
- Never let strangers know that you live alone or are home alone.
- Don't give out personal information to people you don't know.
- If you move to a new home or apartment, change the locks immediately.
- At night, close your curtains or blinds so that no one can see inside your home, and keep your doors and windows locked.
- If you are expecting a service or repair person and are uncomfortable about being alone, ask a friend or relative to be with you during the service call.
- If you have a security system, set it when you leave the house or when you go to bed at night. Memorize your security code and password.
- For your safety and your children's peace of mind, wear a medical-alert device around your neck or on your wrist. If you are in trouble, feeling threatened, ill, or faint, or if you fall, all you have to do is push the button and help will arrive within moments.
- If you're having trouble walking, don't be embarrassed about using a cane or a walker. A choice between accepting the inevitable or taking a bad fall makes the decision pretty obvious. And once you get used to using them, you will feel much steadier and more confident.
- When walking unassisted isn't an option, it's time to consider a wheelchair or a motorized scooter. Both will require an emotional adjustment and a learning curve. Whatever you use, be sure to have the device properly set up by an occupational therapist.

- The use of a mobility aid should not be stigmatized. The best way to dispel negative reactions is to be as comfortable and matter-of-fact as possible. If you are, others will be too.
- Stairs, either inside or outside your home, are accidents waiting to happen. To see steps on a staircase more clearly, alternate each stair with colored carpeting, paint, or strips of tape.

Protect Yourself with an Active Mind and Body

Keeping safe is a do-it-yourself project. While getting older is unavoidable, looking like a frail, little, old person who may fall over in a stiff wind is not. The old saying "move it or lose it" contains much wisdom. Move your body, or your body will lose its ability to do things and take you places. Move your mind, or your mind will simply forget to function.

- Maintain good physical conditioning and fitness. Regular exercise builds muscle tone and endurance and sharpens the mind and senses. Being weak or frail is a serious risk factor.
- Keep moving. Walk as much as possible around the grocery store, to where you park your car, and all over your house. If you're up to it, a regular walking or exercise program is the best present you can give yourself. Working out with a friend is even better.
- To remain healthy and stable, you need to do resistance training to build your strength, cardio exercises to increase your endurance and stamina, and regular stretching to keep you flexible.
- Best of all, exercise is the magic ingredient to improve balance and help prevent falls.
- Exercising the body has a corresponding benefit to the mind. The more you move, the sharper you become. It is even possible to create new brain cells in older people through a process called neuroplasticity (ability of the brain to be flexible and change over the course of a person's lifetime).
- Wear comfortable clothing that does not restrict freedom of movement or your ability to run if that becomes necessary.

- Wear appropriate shoes for exercising. While shoes with shoelaces may all look alike, there are actually different styles for different kinds of exercises.
- If you exercise outside, seek out well-lit, populated areas. If you sense danger, cross the street and head in the opposite direction.
- If you wear a danger-alert button, be prepared to push it at the slightest suspicion of danger.
- If you have a dog, especially a big one, take your loyal companion with you when you exercise outside.
- Don't push yourself to the point of pain. Ignore the advice "no pain, no gain," which is the opposite of smart.

Protect Yourself in Cyberspace

If your parents were reading this book years ago, this section wouldn't have existed. The word cyberspace wouldn't have rung many bells. Nobody was talking about the World Wide Web, the Internet, social media, email, texting, or encrypted passwords. But in the world we live in now, these words are part of our daily lexicon.

- Hard drives die with no warning. Back yours up often.
- If an email asks for your personal information or password, don't give out any information; throw the email in your spam folder.
- Don't believe any email message that tells you have won a lottery or a prize.
- Don't take online or social media quizzes; they are common ways to collect your personal information.
- Lock your mobile phone and your computer and don't give out your password.
- When banking or shopping online, make sure the addresses begin with "https://", which means your data is securely encrypted.
- Don't join unsecured Wi-Fi networks; keep your wireless network password protected.
- Be sure you have security software and keep it up to date.

Protect Yourself from Food Poisoning and Food-Related Risks

If you've ever suffered from food poisoning, you are not likely to forget the experience. Few maladies are more uncomfortable. Sometimes the source is restaurant food, and sometimes it's a meal you prepared at home or ate at a friend's house. Wherever the origin, it provides an unforgettable lesson: Be careful of what you put in your mouth. If you have the slightest suspicion that what you are about to eat seems a little off, politely decline. If you travel to other countries, notorious for getting visitors sick, stick to simple foods and drink bottled water.

- Wash your hands with soap and water before and after handling food.
- Older adults are particularly at risk for developing foodborne illnesses. Make healthy, safe food choices to reduce the chances of becoming ill.
- Avoid raw foods and unpasteurized foods. Keep perishable foods refrigerated at all times.
- Some foods don't mix with medications. When in doubt, consult your pharmacist.
- Stay hydrated; drink six to eight glasses of water a day.
- Check food packaging for expiration dates, and dispose of anything that is expired.
- When in doubt about whether a food is safe, throw it out.
- Follow any special diet your doctor prescribes, and avoid foods that are not on the diet.
- I've recently read many warnings about avoiding sushi and not washing chicken before you cook it. (If these don't make sense to you, check them out with a reputable source before you take any unnecessary chances.)

Protect Yourself Financially

Older people are particularly vulnerable to fraud. Be careful when talking on the phone to people you don't know or being offered a deal that seems too good to be true. If you think you have been targeted, contact your bank immediately.

- Keep your valuable personal possessions, jewelry, important legal papers, cash, securities or bonds in a safety deposit box at the bank or in a secure vault bolted to the floor in your home.
- Don't agree to loans or mortgages without consulting a financial expert or your attorney.
- Don't be pressured into buying any product, enrolling in any services, or making any donations.
- Hang up on telemarketers and block their phone numbers. If you get a call from a company that seems legitimate but they ask you for personal information (like your birth date or Social Security number), hang up.
- Never share any information with companies that call you, even if they claim they are the IRS or a company with which you have an existing business relationship.
- When someone tells you about the latest scam, pay attention and believe it.
- Check your bank statements and charge-account receipts regularly to spot suspicious transactions or purchases you don't remember making.
- Keep a list of all of your accounts and scan your credit cards. File them in your safety deposit box.
- Review your credit reports regularly for any mistakes or irregularities.

Yes, this is a long list, and there are suggestions that may seem over the top or unnecessarily alarmist. As I mentioned at the beginning of this chapter, they may not all be relevant, possible, or necessary—but a little knowledge goes a long way. As I was researching this topic, I was surprised at how many I didn't know or had never thought about. While you may not remember every suggestion in this chapter, just reviewing them on occasion should help you be more alert and aware of potential hazards in the future.

Jonathan Gordon
A Physical Therapist Trained in South Africa

Jonathan Gordon has been a physical therapist for thirty-three years. He studied physical therapy at the University of Capetown in South Africa and earned a master's degree in sports medicine. He immigrated to the United States in 1994, when he recognized the limited future for his family in South Africa and saw a window of opportunity in this country where there was a shortage of physical therapists. He formed a partnership with Jonty Felsher, who was also South African, and began to build Rehabilitation Therapy Services (RPI) into a very successful practice. They now have therapists in twenty-three facilities.

At the beginning of my practice, I dealt mainly with sports injuries and kids. Then I began to treat adults and older adults. My practice right now is mostly seniors, and my whole approach is about what physical therapy can do for them; it's active rather than passive. The question we ask is how can we improve things in spite of structural limitations? We can work on people who have severe problems and see significant improvement in their ability to function. We believe that when you touch a person, you can evaluate his or her physical well-being and produce positive therapeutic results.

When we work with patients, we ask what their goals are. We don't discourage people by telling them their goals are unrealistic or impossible, because we are trying to help them do what they want to do. My philosophy is to focus on how we can enhance patients' abilities and improve their quality of life.

Once we use manual, hands-on techniques in order to reduce muscular dysfunction, we can increase joint range of motion. This decreases pain and improves patients' compliance with their exercise programs. We can introduce exercises, but exercises alone are not enough. We have found this dual approach is very powerful and achieves better long-term results and function.

Something that will seriously reduce that quality of life is falling. Older people who fall more than once or twice are considered fall risks. If you are a fall risk, here are four important questions you should ask yourself:

1. Is your environment designed in a safe way? Are there rugs or other trip hazards on the floor? Is there space to move around with a walker? What can you remove that could pose a problem?

2. Are you stable and balanced on your feet? Should you be wearing sturdier, better-fitting shoes? There are stores that specialize in fitting customers with the right shoes.

3. What kind of adjustments can you make to your surroundings? Do you need better lighting? Maybe you need a stool or a bench across the tub. Stepping over the rim of the bathtub is a risk. If you slip even one time and hit the ground, it can be very dangerous.

4. What is the safest way to do whatever you are doing? That should become your mantra. If you aren't sure, a PT or occupational therapist (OT) can assess your environment, make suggestions, and help you do things more safely.

During the pandemic, we have continued to see patients. We are still touching our patients but being extra cautious, wearing masks and gloves and asking patients to wear masks. I believe the precautions we're taking are keeping everyone safe. We hired an infectious disease doctor to consult with on what to do. We are funded by the government for the next eight weeks. Even though we are seeing fewer patients, we didn't furlough anyone or let anyone go. We are able to pay them their full salary.

We have created a work environment where people are recognized and rewarded. Most of all, we have mutual respect. We involve everyone in decisions and communicate changes effectively and openly with therapists and those who work out front and in back offices. We encourage their input and respect their opinions. This is a good place to work—a fun, comfortable environment.

In a lot of practices people are given unrealistic expectations, such as having to see too many patients in too short a time. We don't operate that way. I work with our physical therapists, and we do a lot of peer-to-peer training. We believe that being in a healthy place creates healthy people. The biggest thing we do is practice what we preach. When employees see the leadership behaving in a certain way, they follow suit. When I am treating patients, I work side by side with our PTs and physical therapy assistants (PTAs). I am not the boss. I am one of them.

IV. TURNING IN YOUR CAR KEYS

When is the right time to stop driving?

HOW MANY TIMES have you found yourself on a highway, stuck behind a car going ten miles below the speed limit, only to discover that the driver was a little, old person who could barely see over the steering wheel? And how many times have you thought he or she was an accident waiting to happen? How many times (if at all) has it occurred to you that *you* are holding up traffic on a highway or busy street because you're driving too slowly? None of us wants to believe we are that little, old person, but it may be time to ask yourself if you are being unusually cautious on the road or the subject of unfriendly looks from other drivers.

According to the AAA Foundation for Traffic Safety, by the year 2031, one in every five drivers in America will be sixty-five years of age or older. As older drivers, we possess a wide range of abilities; yet some of us have bought into the misconception that we pose a risk to ourselves and others on the road. One of our greatest strengths is experience, and experience does not decline with age. However, some skills necessary for safe driving, such as vision, reflexes, flexibility, and hearing do begin to deteriorate, and we need to recognize when they do.

Few of us at any age are very good at assessing how well we drive. With no objective evaluation, we feel pretty confident about our driving.

The AAA Foundation for Traffic Safety provides a self-rating form to take the guesswork out of assessing when it's time to stop driving.

Here are some specific questions on the form that have concrete answers: How many traffic tickets, warnings, or "discussions" with traffic police have you had in the past two years? How many accidents (major or minor) have you had, and have your insurance rates increased as a result? Have your children or other family members expressed concern about your driving habits, and have you become defensive when they did? If you are piling up traffic tickets or repair bills, it's hard to deny their existence.

How up to date are you on changes in driving and traffic laws? Do you have any idea how your medications affect your driving? How often do you get your eyes checked? And what about your behavior behind the wheel? Most of us wear our seatbelts, but do you signal and check your rear and side-view mirrors when you change lanes? Did you even know you are supposed to do that?

And, finally, do you become impatient with other drivers or flustered when other drivers are impatient with you? Are you uneasy at busy intersections or when you're merging onto a highway, or do you find yourself avoiding highways altogether?

If these questions make you uncomfortable, I can assure you they had the same effect on me. My car had a built-in safety package that let me know when I had wandered out of my lane or should have slowed down before I was ready to plow into the car in front of me. I remember when my mother had a string of small accidents, and my sister had the unpleasant task of taking away her car keys—something I did not want to experience. When I stopped driving, I wanted it to be my decision.

I must admit that when I contemplated all the losses that come with aging, the one I feared most was losing my car. The car has always been a necessity for me because St. Louis lags well behind other major cities with its public transportation. But I also knew that if I needed an item from Walgreens, I could jump in the car and be there in two minutes. A car represented much more than transportation: it was freedom, autonomy, and status. One doesn't give up those things easily.

Since my "bad driving" was frequently brought to my attention, I had been pondering this inevitable moment of letting go. This would not be an easy decision, but someday it *was* going to happen. Someday came sooner than I had anticipated. Of all the reasons I've listed above, the most persuasive was my doctor's suggestion that I stop driving. In my family, much research and price comparison precede every big decision. That's why the speed with which this one was made and implemented made my head spin.

I drove to the Honda dealer to track down the person in charge of used-car sales, who had been unavailable for three days. When the leasing manager walked by, I stopped him and explained what I was trying to do and why. He said, "Okay, I'll take care of it."

And take care of it he did—in record time. I signed all the papers, cleaned out any personal items still in my car, handed in my keys, and walked away—free and clear—*owing not one penny*. Honda had bought back the car and assumed the lease (They loved the fact that the car had fewer than twelve thousand miles). It was a done deal.

However, as Alan Alda said in *Same Time Next Year*, "I guess I didn't think it through." Deciding how I would get from one place to another should definitely have been step one in this process—and then selling the car as step two. I did it backwards, leaving me with no transportation and no plan. Obviously, there are a few flaws in this approach. While most big cities have public transportation and people are accustomed to using it, my hometown is a little behind the times.

A few years ago, there would have been practically no options except cabs and begging rides. But now we have the miracle of Lyft, Uber, and a host of other ways to get around. What follows are five affordable senior transportation options:

1. Most counties across the United States offer free or low-cost public transportation services designed for seniors who need door-to-door

rides. The best way to find these programs is to call your county's **Area Agency on Aging.** They'll connect you with available local programs. The **ElderCareLocator** is another way to find local government transportation programs. Just enter your zip code in the search box at the top of the page.

2. **GoGoGrandparent** is a concierge service that connects seniors with on-demand ride services like Lyft and Uber. These services can have a car at your location in minutes and are best for seniors who are able to get in and out of a vehicle without assistance. Riders pay the regular price for the on-demand ride plus an additional fee for the concierge service. On-demand ride fares vary but are generally lower than taxi rates.

3. **Lyft** is a popular on-demand ride service that provides transportation quickly. It is best for independent seniors who are comfortable using smartphone apps and can get in and out of a car without assistance. Concierge service (no smartphone required) is available through such Lyft partners as assisted living communities, health organizations, etc. Ask local organizations if they partner with Lyft.

4. **Veyo** is a company that partners with insurance companies and health facilities to provide non-emergency medical transportation covered as an insurance benefit. Veyo is appropriate for seniors who need transportation to medical appointments or a specialized vehicle to accommodate a wheelchair or stretcher. The service is free if the health facility's insurance company offers Veyo as a transportation benefit.

5. **ITNAmerica** is a national network of senior-ride-companies that offer door-*through*-door transportation. The number of locations is limited, but it's a great option if available in your area. It is best for those who need assistance in and out of the car and through the door of their destination. Rates are affordable, but pricing varies depending on the local affiliate.

Some of these services may not be offered in your community, and others may be strictly local. Most charge a fee, but compared to owning a car or taking cabs, they are less expensive. I decided to investigate further. After trying out Lyft and GoGoGrandparent, I went back to Google to find out what else was available in my area. Here is what I found:

1. **Aging Ahead (1-800-243-6060):** There is an area agency on aging in every county in the United States. The advantage is that it is a free service, though contributions are welcome. The disadvantage is that you must call someone who will come out and register you, and they require three or four days' notice to set up a ride.

2. **The St. Louis County Older Residents' Program (CORP) (314-615-4516):** This appears to be part of the Aging Ahead program described above. Disadvantages are that there seems to be a long wait time to set up a ride, but you could call the day before to see what's available.

3. **The Magic Bus (314-581-4842):** The advantage is that you can make reservations for three trips. Any area resident with a disability or age sixty and above is eligible, and you can book regular rides. The disadvantages are that it only services communities nearby; and riders must not have any conditions that require special handling, medical attention, or any condition that might adversely affect the health of other participants in the vehicle. This is obviously a specialized service for a particular neighborhood, but there may be others like it elsewhere.

4. **ITNGateway (636-329-0888):** St. Charles, Missouri, or (314-724-2117) St. Louis, Missouri. This is a national organization with two locations set up in the St. Louis area. Based on my experience so far, this is my favorite.

Getting the Facts

Important decisions, such as whether to stop driving, should be made based on knowing the facts. Yes, your feelings and emotions are important, but if you stubbornly insist on doing something that is not in your best interest, deep down you know it's the wrong thing to do. Here are some irrefutable facts; any decision you make should take these facts into consideration.

- As you age, your vision, reflexes, and hearing change; these changes can make it harder for you to drive safely.
- People age seventy and older are more likely to crash than any other age group besides those twenty-five and younger. And because older drivers are more fragile, they are more likely to get hurt or die in these crashes.
- There is no set age when people should stop driving. Each person is different, but keep in mind that most people drive seven to ten years longer than they should. Here are some warning signs to watch for:
  » You are nervous or frightened when you drive.
  » Other drivers often honk at you.
  » You have trouble staying in your lane.
  » You get lost, even on roads you know.
  » You are driving slower than other drivers around you.
  » You frequently miss your turn or exit.
  » You are unsure of yourself behind the wheel.
  » You start having accidents, even if they are only fender benders.
  » You are worried about getting into a more serious car crash.
  » You are afraid your driving might lead to someone else getting hurt.
  » Your family is worried about your driving.
  » You have stiffness or joint pain that makes turning your head or the steering wheel difficult.
  » You have problems seeing or hearing clearly.

What You Should Do

- Be honest with yourself about whether any of the above warning signs hit home. If any do, consider turning in your car keys.

- Take a driver-safety course for older drivers to objectively measure how well you drive.

The Benefits of Not Driving

- Obviously, the first is that you are safer if you stop driving when all indications are that you should.
- Believe it or not, another of the benefits is a sense of relief. You may not even realize that you are stressed when you drive until the feeling is no longer present.
- There is satisfaction in knowing that you are no longer putting yourself, your passengers, other drivers, or pedestrians at risk.

When to Stop Driving

I have heard it said that older people self-monitor, and when we realize we're having trouble doing something, we stop. No one has to tell us that night driving is getting harder. Oncoming lights are blinding, street signs are invisible, and it's difficult to judge how close we are to the car in front of us. The problem with driving in bad weather—rain or snow—is twofold: Sometimes it was hard for me to see two feet in front of my car, even if I was handling the road pretty well. Often other drivers create a bigger hazard than the weather. We know when it's time to stop. *I* certainly knew, but it took a firm suggestion from my doctor to spur me into action.

Vicki Spraul
President and founder of Gray Matters Alliance (GMA)

Vicki Spraul is the president and founder of Gray Matters Alliance (GMA), an organization dedicated to keeping aging and intellectually and developmentally disabled adults safe at home and on the roads. She also serves as a facilitator for Keeping Us Safe's self-assessment program for older drivers, a valuable tool for helping older people and their families make appropriate decisions about their ability to drive safely. Vicki is a recipient of the Bill and Betty Fresch Outstanding Achievement Award for demonstrating unwavering dedication and compassion in helping older adults.

◆　◆　◆

I established Gray Matters Alliance about six years ago because of my love of seniors. I started out doing empathy workshops to give people an idea of the limitations that come with getting old—maybe stiff fingers, poor eyesight, longer reaction time, or trouble buttoning up a shirt. I put able-bodied people through a live, interactive workshop. It was great except I wasn't dealing with any seniors, and that's what I like to do.

A few years ago, I met a gentleman who started a company that gives enhanced self-assessments to seniors. I am licensed to administer these assessments. There are probably about seventy or eighty people like me across the country who do the same thing. We try to help the families that are having problems with a family member who doesn't want to stop driving. We assess whether that person should continue to drive or stop.

We go to the older person's home, so he doesn't have to come to us. We like to do it right at the kitchen table. We will spend a couple of hours with that person and try to get an idea of his activity level and what medications he is taking. In between those learning conversations, we do some very simple paper-and-pencil cognitive exercises. One is the clock test (a fast, simple way of spotting warning signs for Alzheimer's disease and other dementias that can be administered by non-professionals), and we do some roadside-sign recognition.

Then, if we think it's safe enough, we'll go for a ride in the person's own car because that's what he's comfortable with, as opposed to a clinic car or a simulator. What we're trying to do through that whole session is to discover why the older person doesn't want to give up the keys and whether he even needs to. The common thread among their reasons seems to be their independence and what is at the other end of their drive. Are they going to pick up prescriptions, attend a card game, play Mah-jongg, or have lunch with friends? These are the things they think they're going to lose.

We provide workbooks for families, conduct family empowerment classes, and work with adult children. Parents often have trouble with their children's emotions and opinions, but when a third-party works with them, we don't have the history or know what buttons to push as the children do. Sometimes adult siblings aren't on the same page, and the older person pits one child against the other. We try to keep emotion and opinions out of it and just stick to the facts.

When we meet with the family, we ask questions like, *Where does your mom like to go? Does she have a standard beauty shop appointment? Where does your dad like to go? How often does he go there? If he had to find an alternate ride, does he have one?* If the answer is yes, we know they have thought it out. If the answer is no, we have to figure out a way to get Dad from point A (his home) to point B (his destination). Is it Call a Ride? Is it a transportation service here in town? Is it Lyft or Uber? Is it going to be a family member?. We want to have those how-am-I-going-to-get-there questions answered.

Finding alternate forms of transportation is the key. When we follow up on people whom we advised not to drive, we find that Mom is more social than she used to be. It's because Mom has figured out how to call for rides, or the rides are set up for her; and she's going out more than she would if she had to drive herself. She doesn't have to worry about the rain or the snow or finding a parking spot, and when she gives in to the fact that someone else is going to drive her, it's no big deal. And it's actually even better because it's door-to-door service.

When we do our sessions, the ultimate goal is for the individuals to come to their own conclusions that maybe they don't drive as well as they used to and finally agree to stop. We want older adults to be more self-aware. We want them to recognize that their reaction time is slower or cars are darting out in front of them. We do encounter people who dig in their heels and just keep driving, or they say they will stop but then sneak out and drive. We make our recommendation, but it's actually the family's decision. Or a physician or the state or law enforcement may have to step in.

When I first started, I was surprised to get calls from individuals who wanted to know if they should be driving. Sometimes it's just a matter of wanting to get a son or daughter off their backs. Or maybe they just got out of rehab after a stroke and they want to be sure that they're OK to drive because they don't want to put anyone in danger. Or it may be that their doctor won't release them until they have their driving assessed. Sometimes I don't recommend that they stop driving altogether but only that they limit their driving: Don't drive in rush hour, don't drive on highways, don't drive at night or when it's raining.

Every individual is different, so our approach is case by case. Maybe the issue is stability, maybe it's cognitive, or maybe the person has had a stroke or a traumatic brain injury. Some people live in rural areas and can't get rides easily. Others live in the city and have used public transportation all their lives. Some have always been self-reliant and aren't used to getting rides.

Sometimes a person can still drive, but the family sees signs that down the road he isn't going to be able to. During that interim, while the person is still driving, it's a good idea to try out alternate forms of transportation and not wait until this situation comes to a complete halt.

We want older people to be empowered. By the time individuals have to stop driving, they may have already lost their health or a spouse or a pet or the home they've lived in for forty years. Giving up the car is the last in a long line of losses. We try to give them a choice.

V. STAYING HEALTHY

What will it take to maintain your vigor and vitality?

AS WE GET OLDER, THE LIST OF THINGS we might worry about seems to grow by the day. Will I run out of money? Will I be alone without friends, family, or a support system? Will I develop Alzheimer's? Will I be safe in my home? Will my health deteriorate? Not everyone worries about the same aspects of aging; we each have our own Achilles heel. Mine happens to be health—mental and physical. If my mind stops working, how will I continue to write, which has been my *raison d'être* for my entire adult life? If my body breaks down, how can I remain independent and mobile?

Here are two things I know: (1) Human beings age, and as we do, inevitable changes take place in our bodies; and (2) Some of these changes are out of our control. They are simply part of being human. On the other hand, we do have the power to slow down or even prevent some of the diseases and changes in how we look and feel. The more we understand about our own bodies and what they need, the better able we will be to live long and healthy lives. Scientific studies have revealed that the human body self-destructs as we age, but the speed at which it breaks down is up to us. The opposite of early self-destruction is healthy aging.

What *Is* Healthy Aging?

Technically, healthy aging is being free of disease, functioning at a high physical and cognitive level, and being socially engaged and productive. According to Dr. Andrew Weil, a well-known American doctor who promotes a holistic approach to medicine, "Although aging is an irreversible process, there are myriad things you can do to keep your mind and body in good working order through all phases of your life. Aging doesn't have to mean you have to get old in the process. You can stay attractive, healthy looking, enthusiastic, and energetic. Your daily routines affect every aspect of your life from the firmness of your skin to the sharpness of your mind. No matter how old you are or what your physical condition is, if you want to change, start where you are right now."

Here are five suggestions for how to begin.

1. First and foremost, take care of yourself. Self-care includes doing whatever you can to minimize your stress and stay positive. We all know that stress and negativity play havoc with our immune systems and are linked to many serious medical conditions.

2. Do the basics: Stay away from junk food; eat fruits, vegetables, and protein; drink plenty of water; and get adequate sleep. If you don't need as much sleep as you did when you were younger, that's normal, but at least try to rest when you are tired.

3. Do whatever you can to help others, even if it's just a phone call to say hi. I am reading a book called *29 Gifts: How a Month of Giving Can Change Your Life*, and I'm discovering how many ways there are to give—even if you're housebound.

4. Stay in touch with people. Solitude is lovely, but isolation can be lonely. If you are computer literate, you can communicate with friends and family on social media, FaceTime, Skype, or Zoom, which is the newest vehicle for reaching out to touch somebody. If you are not comfortable using electronic devices, this might be a great time

to learn. Enlist the help of a grandchild if you have one, to teach you the fundamentals.

5. Feed your creative side. Dust off your paints or gel pens and create art; lose yourself in sewing or knitting; practice piano; plant a garden, inside or outside; keep a journal; or write letters to the editor or to your senators and representatives. If you have always wanted to write a book, this would be a perfect time to start.

Other Concerns, Other Cautions

Before the pandemic captured the world's attention, you were probably aware of some of the chronic conditions that plague older people. You may have even experienced some of them first-hand.

- **Arthritis** is probably the number-one condition that affects people sixty-five and older. The CDC estimates that close to 50 percent of all adults over that age have some kind of painful arthritis.
- **Heart disease** remains the leading killer of older adults. As you age, you tend to live with risk factors, such as high blood pressure and high cholesterol, that increase your chances of developing heart disease or having a stroke.
- **Cancer** is the second leading cause of death among people over age sixty-five, striking an average of 25 percent of seniors. The good news is that it can be caught early through mammograms, colonoscopies, and skin checks; and many types of cancer are treatable.
- **Respiratory diseases,** such as chronic obstructive pulmonary disease (COPD), are the third most common cause of death among seniors. An average of 11 percent of the population has asthma, chronic bronchitis, or emphysema and is vulnerable to pneumonia and other infections.
- **Alzheimer's disease** was found in 11 percent of older people several years ago, according to the Alzheimer's Association, but because diagnosis is challenging, it's difficult to know exactly how many people are living with this chronic condition.

- **Osteoporosis** affects 54 million Americans over age fifty, putting them at risk for a fracture, decreasing their mobility, and sometimes leading to disability, reports the National Osteoporosis Foundation.
- **Diabetes** affects an estimated 25 percent of people over sixty-five and caused more than 54 thousand deaths in 2014. Notes the CDC, diabetes can be identified and treated early with simple blood tests for blood sugar levels.
- **Influenza and pneumonia** aren't chronic conditions but are among the top eight causes of death in older people. Seniors are more vulnerable to these diseases and less able to fight them off.
- **Falls** that require emergency-room care increase with age. Most falls occur in the home, where tripping hazards include area rugs and slippery bathroom floors.
- **Substance abuse** and alcohol abuse are a concern because of possible interactions with prescription medication and their impact on seniors' overall health.
- **Obesity** is an important health-risk factor for heart disease, diabetes, and cancer—all chronic conditions that have an impact on quality of life. As the numbers on the scale increase, so does the risk for disease.
- **Depression** has afflicted 15 to 20 percent of Americans over sixty-five, according to the American Psychological Association. Depression can lower immunity and compromise your ability to fight infections.
- **Healthy teeth and gums** are important not just for a pretty smile and easy eating, but also for your overall health. As you age, your mouth tends to become dryer, and cavities are more difficult to prevent. According to the CDC, 25 percent of adults over sixty-five have no natural teeth.
- **Poverty** affects seniors when they are unable to afford doctor visits, medication for chronic conditions, and other essential healthcare needs. Older women are slightly more likely than men to be living in poverty, and that gap widens in those over eighty.

- **Shingles** is the adult version of chicken pox. According to the National Institutes of Health, one out of three people over sixty will get shingles, and 50 percent of all Americans will experience it before they are eighty.

It is not my intention to make you throw up your hands in despair. Many of these conditions can be prevented by making a few sensible changes to your lifestyle. What you eat and whether you smoke are certainly within your control. While there isn't much you can do about heredity, you can choose to exercise, get regular cancer screenings, have routine dental checkups and bone density tests, avail yourself of annual flu shots and pneumonia and shingles vaccines, monitor your alcohol intake and your use of recreational drugs, and seek help if you are depressed.

Even if you do everything you can to protect your health and avoid some of these debilitating conditions, you may find yourself living with one or more of them as you age. Living with chronic medical conditions is never easy and even less so when that condition is invisible, which means it isn't as apparent on the surface as it would be if you were walking around with a cast on your arm or using crutches. According to research, 96 percent of people in the United States who have chronic medical conditions show no outward signs of their illness, and 10 percent experience disabling symptoms. It is estimated that one in ten people lives with an invisible disability.

Understanding the Changes that Come with Age

What follows is a long list of possible changes to your body, how they may affect you as you age, and what you can do to prevent or minimize them. You are unlikely to experience all of them, but remember, knowledge is power. The more you know, the better able you will be to maintain your health, vitality, and independence.

Some of these changes are subtle and not immediately observable, such as those having to do with digestive health. If you are prone to

81

indigestion or have ulcers, no one has to know except your doctor. Others are more obvious, such as walking more slowly and forgetting people's names. Neither of these are cause for concern, but when the changes begin to add up, you may begin to wonder if what you are going through is normal.

You May Experience:
- Changes in the texture of your skin and hair
- Loss of calcium, minerals, and bone mass or density—particularly in women past menopause
- The need for fewer calories but the same or greater amount of nutrients
- Changes in your joints
- Increased risk of vitamin B12 deficiency
- Becoming particularly prone to dehydration due to lack of thirst
- Loss of function in your kidneys
- Decreased appetite—hungry less often and feeling full more quickly
- Diminished sense of smell and taste
- Unintended weight loss and nutritional deficiencies

The Effects of These Changes:
- Bones become more brittle and may break more easily.
- Overall height decreases.
- Joint changes range from minor stiffness to severe arthritis.
- Posture may become more stooped (bent).
- Knees and hips may become more flexed.
- The neck may tilt, and the shoulders may narrow, while the pelvis becomes wider.
- Movement slows and becomes limited.
- Walking may become unsteady with less arm swinging.
- Having less energy may lead to feeling fatigued more often.
- Strength and endurance diminish.

- Loss of muscle mass reduces strength.
- Reflexes are reduced due to changes in the muscles and tendons.
- Inability to move on your own or stretch muscles with exercise may produce muscle contractures.

How to Prevent or Reduce These Changes

- Exercise is one of the best ways to slow or prevent problems with the muscles, joints, and bones. A moderate exercise program can help you maintain strength, balance, and flexibility. Exercise helps the bones stay strong. (More on this in the next section).
- Eat a well-balanced diet with plenty of calcium. Women need to be particularly careful to get enough calcium and vitamin D as they age. Post-menopausal women and men over age seventy should take in 1,200 mg of calcium per day. Women and men over age seventy should get 800 international units (IU) of vitamin D daily.
- If you have osteoporosis, talk to your physician about prescription treatments.
- Eat nutrient-rich, whole foods.
- Increase fiber intake to protect against bowel-related issues, including constipation and diverticulitis.
- Take a vitamin B12 supplement or consume foods fortified with vitamin B12.
- Eat a diet rich in fruits, vegetables, fish, and lean meats to obtain potassium, omega-3 fatty acids, magnesium, and iron.
- Stay hydrated. Make a conscious effort to drink enough water daily. If you find drinking water a challenge, as I do, try having one to two glasses of water with each meal, or carry a water bottle with you during the day.
- Divide your meals into smaller portions, eat every few hours, or eat healthy snacks, such as almonds, yogurt, and hard-boiled eggs, which provide lots of nutrients and calories.

The Value of Exercise

A few years ago when I was working on another project, I came across a book called *Spark: The Revolutionary New Science of Exercise and the Brain* by John J. Ratey, MD and Eric Hagerman. *Spark* is the first book to explore the connection between exercise and the brain. In it, Dr. Ratey presents startling research to prove that exercise is truly our best defense against everything from depression to ADD to addiction to aggression to menopause to Alzheimer's. I could not put this book down.

According to the author, "Exercise can help you beat stress, lift your mood, fight memory loss, sharpen your intellect, and function better than ever simply by elevating your heart rate and breaking a sweat." The evidence is undeniable: Aerobic exercise physically restructures our brains for peak performance. Cognitive decline in older people is not a given. In the chapter on aging, Dr. Ratey explains that exercise may not only stop brain cells from dying but actually help to develop new brain cells.

Why We Need Each Other

John Donne's poem, "No Man is an Island," has particular meaning for older people. Human beings don't do well when we are isolated from others; we need to be part of a community in order to thrive. The third level of Abraham Maslow's hierarchy of needs is *belonging*. We need each other. We grow up in tribes and families. All through our lives we make friends. We socialize with neighbors and people with whom we have something in common, such as our religious or political leanings. We work with others towards shared economic goals. We play on sports teams or spend time with other parents watching our children play. Throughout life, close friends provide a strong foundation of compassion and trust for many people, and they can become even more important as we age.

But as the years go by, our community shrinks. When we retire, we lose touch with former work colleagues and friends. Loved ones may move away. We experience the death of friends and family members. And often we find ourselves living alone. The loss of social support plays a significant role in our overall health as we age.

Spending time with friends and family members can boost your quality of life, including both physical and mental health. For older people, developing various positive sources of social support reduces stress, wards off anxiety and depression, and reduces the risk of some physical health conditions.

We are becoming more aware of how social interactions can affect cognitive health. Researchers have long known about the health benefits of what is known as "social capital"—the ties that build trust, connection, and participation. But this link may be particularly important for seniors, precisely because both our health and our social capital tend to decline as we age.

One study found that cognitive abilities decline much more slowly in individuals who have frequent social connections compared to those who have little social contact with others. Socialization has other benefits as well. It may improve memory and longevity as it reduces stress and isolation. Many older people socialize by spending time in group exercise classes, which can provide a number of physical benefits, including the potential to increase lifespan.

Keeping Your Brain Busy

Everyone has lapses in memory from time to time, but significant memory loss is not a normal part of getting older. It's important to talk with your doctor if you are experiencing memory loss and other cognitive symptoms that interfere with normal activities and relationships. Before you panic, you should know that promising research indicates that taking the following steps can help keep your mind sharp as you age:

- **Control cholesterol problems and high blood pressure.** Cardiovascular health—having healthy blood sugar, cholesterol levels, and blood pressure—is associated with better cognitive function.

- **Don't smoke or drink excessively.** Because these are both seen as putting you at increased risk for dementia, kick the habit if you smoke, and if you drink, cut back on the amount you consume.
- **Exercise regularly.** I know I've covered this in depth, but you should know that consistent, vigorous exercise helps maintain blood flow to the brain and lower the risk of dementia, according to a study published in the *Annals of Medicine* in 2015.
- **Be aware of what you are eating.** Vitamin E, B vitamins, and Omega-3 fatty acids along with avoiding saturated fat could help prevent dementia, according to an article published in 2016 in the *Annals of the New York Academy of Sciences.*
- **Become a lifelong learner.** People with more years of formal education are at lower risk for Alzheimer's and other dementias than those with fewer years of formal education, according to the Alzheimer's Association. Education is not limited to four years of college between the ages of eighteen and twenty-two. Growing numbers of older adults do go back to school or sign up for lifelong learning programs at local universities.
- **Stimulate your brain.** You can also keep your mind active by learning new skills. A 2017 study published in *The American Journal of Geriatric Psychiatry* suggests that acquiring skills in later life, including those related to adopting new technologies, may have the potential to reduce or delay cognitive changes associated with aging.
- **Socialize more.** Making new friends or spending time with the ones you have might be good for your brain. A 2018 study published in *Scientific Reports* that looked at older adults in China found that participants with consistently high or increased social engagement had a lower risk of dementia than those with consistently low social engagement.
- **You are what you eat.** According to the "Dietary Guidelines for Americans, Key Recommendations for Older Adults (US Dept. of

Agriculture, 2010), older people who are well and active for their age and do not have any major diseases should follow these guidelines:

» Reduce your calorie intake over time without reducing your nutrient intake. Consume enough energy (calories) to maintain a healthy weight throughout life.

» Limit your intake of sodium, refined grains, solid fats, and added sugar, particularly liquid sugar in sweetened cold drinks and undiluted fruit juices.

» Increase physical activity and spend less time being sedentary.

» Get enough protein. Unless you have problems with your kidneys or diabetes, a slightly higher protein level should help you to maintain lean muscle mass.

» Eat nutrient-dense foods and drink nutrient-dense beverages.

» Select fat-free or low-fat milk and milk products (yogurt, cottage cheese) to boost calcium intake, maintain healthy bones, and prevent osteoporosis.

» Incorporate seafood, lean meats, poultry, and eggs into your diet to boost your high-quality protein, as well as vitamin B12, iron, and trace minerals, such as zinc and selenium.

» Include dried beans, peas, lentils, and soy products as an excellent source of dietary fiber, vitamins, minerals, and plant protein.

» Eat vegetables as often as possible, particularly dark green or dark yellow vegetables, which are rich in beta-carotene (e.g., spinach, butternut squash, pumpkin, sweet potatoes, peas).

» Try to eat at least 50 percent of all grains as whole grains (i.e., high-fiber breakfast cereals, wholegrain breads, rolls, and biscuits).

» Eat real foods, rather than liquid meal supplements, although these are helpful if you have problems with eating or need to gain weight.

» Use alcohol in moderation—no more than one or two drinks per day and not necessarily every day. Alcohol should never take the place of nutrient-dense foods or drinks, such as milk.

» If you struggle to eat a balanced diet, you may benefit from taking a multivitamin and mineral supplement, a calcium supplement, and salmon oil capsules to boost Omega-3 intake.

» The use of probiotics ("good or beneficial microorganisms") can benefit people of all ages, especially older people.

» If you look at ads in magazines or commercials for dating sites, you will get Madison Avenue's version of what you should look like. It would seem that every older person (you can tell they're older because they have gray hair) is attractive, active, and slim. They are all paired off with equally appealing significant others, or they are surrounded by friends of approximately the same age who are full of energy and enthusiasm. This isn't too surprising, since at every age both men and women are presented in the way we would all like to look.

But let's get real; most of us don't come close to that ideal. We do what we can to look our very best, but two factors play a role in the image we present to the world. The first one, which is pretty much out of our hands, is heredity. If your parents were movie-star gorgeous, chances are they passed along some of those genes to you. The second is the inner glow of vitality that results from a healthy lifestyle. If you really are what you eat, chances are you tend to have a salad for lunch as opposed to a Big Mac and fries. And if exercise is the secret of good health, lacing up your running shoes rather than firing up the sports network would seem to be a better choice.

Monique Williams, MD
A Geriatrician with a Leading Hospital System

Dr. Monique M. Williams is a geriatrician in St. Louis, Missouri. She has been in practice more than eleven years and specializes in the unique

health needs of the elderly, including chronic diseases, nutritional prob-
lems, skin ailments, cognitive loss, memory impairment, adverse effects
of medications, immobility and balances issues. She works with patients,
their families, and medical specialists to coordinate care.

◆ ◆ ◆

There is a difference between a gerontologist and a geriatrician. Gerontology is the study of the science of aging; geriatrics focuses on caring for older people.

One important role geriatricians play is educating patients and their families about aging and how to practice preventive healthcare. We talk to our patients and try to determine their stressors and issues. Caring for an older patient is a family affair, but adult children may not agree with what their parent wants to do. We advise patients to bring a family member to doctor's visits.

Geriatricians take a holistic approach to each patient. We can see the big picture and often spot the early stages of a problem. At that point, we will refer the patient to the correct specialist—a pulmonologist if it is a lung issue, a rheumatologist if she suspects arthritis, or a neurologist for early onset dementia or neuropathy.

Older adults may have multiple conditions and see a specialist for each one. Geriatricians work with these specialists to coordinate care. Basically, I act as a quarterback for the medical team. Electronic health records (EHR) help by making information about each patient available across the hospital system.

Given the rising tide of people over the age of sixty-five, *poly-pharmacy*—taking multiple medications or more than are medically necessary—is a growing concern in older adults who are at the highest risk of adverse effects. It's important to know what medications the patient is taking. If prescriptions are usually filled at the same drugstore, the pharmacy department will keep a database of past and present prescriptions.

The most important piece of advice I can offer my patients is to think about your goals and objectives in terms of your quality of life. What is your priority? Make your own decisions. We are changing perceptions of aging in this country. The trend is toward patient-centered care, with patients involved in decision-making. It is important to have family discussions where older people can openly express their feelings and desires. You need to talk about advanced-care planning—how you wish to be cared for in your later years. You can't just leave the subject to chance. These are not easy conversations to have, and they can become quite emotional. Adult children should not feel that they are parenting their parents; rather, they are offering suggestions and support.

One of the issues today is whether older adults have sufficient access to the physicians they need. There are not enough geriatricians for our rapidly aging population. Compared to other specialties, this one doesn't seem very exciting. By the time they get to middle school, kids find high-tech more appealing than high touch. That's why we have to start talking about caring for older people when children are very young—to get them used to the idea.

(For additional information on geriatrics and geriatricians, visit the National Institute on Aging website at www.nia.nih.gov.)

Diana Gates*
Lifelong Exerciser

Diana Gates is a retired psychotherapist who practiced in agency settings and private practice for forty-six years. No matter what has gone on in her life, including working two or three jobs at a time, numerous car accidents, and a debilitating autoimmune disorder, she just kept working on her health—exercising and eating well. No matter how bad she felt or how tired she was, she knew what she had to do to stay well, and as much as she was able to, she just did it. Now, in her early seventies, Diana is retired and pursuing all of the activities she loves, from reading long-neglected books to taking piano lessons. And she is still exercising, cooking healthy foods, and getting plenty of rest.

*Name has been changed to protect the interviewee's identity.

◆ ◆ ◆

When I was younger, I thought I'd be able to work indefinitely as a licensed clinical social worker. I thought that as long as I could listen closely to people, understand them, provide feedback, and counsel, I could continue to function as a psychotherapist. And I certainly committed myself to staying abreast of evolving therapies, including becoming a certified Eye Movement Desensitization and Reprocessing (EMDR) therapist and consultant.

I wanted to assertively take care of my body and avoid health issues. As a young person, I thought that if I took care of myself and ate properly, my health would always be good. I think I always knew I would eat well and exercise. Meditation was a part of it, though I wasn't a regular meditator. There was something about mindfulness that really attracted me. I always cooked, even as a child, and that continued into adulthood. Cooking lends itself to healthy eating.

As I moved past sixty, each year of work became more difficult, leaving me exhausted not only at the end of the day, but midway through the day. I realized that I had pushed my limits by working two and sometimes three jobs through quite a few years of my career.

All the while, I was experiencing chronic pain as a result of twelve auto accidents and fatigue due to an auto-immune disorder that was diagnosed some twenty-odd years ago. Most of the auto accidents were when someone rear-ended my car, and there was whiplash each time, which really took a toll on me. So, why do I have headaches? Why do I have multilevel degenerative disc disease? It was because of all those car accidents that just kept happening.

Exercise was something I tried to incorporate into my life; some years I did well, and other years I failed miserably. Swing dancing, swimming, yoga, tai chi, bicycling, and walking were all parts of my exercise regimen at different times. However, often those activities were relegated to the weekends (which did not serve me well) because of my long hours and fatigue. After the multiple car accidents, pain management was part of the balancing act for me, so I also sought help from meditation practices and various physical treatments to manage pain.

In 1990, I started my private practice, which I worked at full-time until 1997, when managed care more or less knocked a hole in most private practices. From 1990 to 1997, I had health insurance through the National Organization of Women (NOW), but that insurance became unaffordable. So, I knew I had to get back into agency or hospital work in order to have health insurance. That's when I went to Chestnut Health Systems, an agency in Illinois, and managed their outpatient mental health program from 1997 to 2007.

Initially I worked full-time, but eventually I was able to cut back to part-time because I continued to see clients in my private practice. The agency wanted me to work full-time, so I started looking for jobs in St. Louis to avoid the commute to Illinois. From 2007 to 2015, I worked for a St. Louis-based, family-service agency as manager of clinical services. Sometimes I felt my management work was easier than my clinical practice.

As I moved towards sixty-six, I was working thirty-two hours a week as a manager and approximately twenty to twenty-five hours a week in my private practice. I thought I could manage (and at first, I did) to balance the management work with private practice because I had done that type of juggling act for quite a few years. To me, the management work was usually less draining than the clinical work. However, at some point I was tired of being "sandwiched" between trying to advocate for my staff (and the clients they served) and the overwhelming demands of the upper-echelon management of the agency.

In late 2014, I had a knee replacement and was off work for about six weeks. I returned to work in late January 2015. I thought I could manage but soon realized that, between the continued rehab for my knee and two jobs, something had to give. The pivotal day was a day when both the executive director and my immediate supervisor told me that I was to take on a caseload of clients at the agency in addition to my management and supervisory responsibilities. Fortunately, I was already on Medicare, so I didn't need their health insurance plan anymore. I had also paid off my mortgage and was able to resign and turn my attention solely to my private practice.

Once I left the agency work, I did focus on my private practice and determined that a caseload of fifteen clients per week was my maximum, in terms of my energy. I worked about that number of hours per week, plus about another five hours on paperwork and administrative tasks. I tried to establish a consistent exercise schedule, starting with water exercise classes. By May, I graduated to yoga classes and walking. Throughout this time, and continuing to the present, I received regular physical therapy.

My husband was a chiropractor, and for most of our marriage he would frequently adjust me so I could go to work. But as soon as I was eligible for Medicare, I started to look into other options because it is stressful for a healthcare professional to treat his or her family members. By that point, I was working fewer hours and didn't have to have work done every day. I could see my chiropractor once or twice a week, and that would be sufficient.

Even after improvements with strengthening exercises, I continued to experience a high level of fatigue, feeling as though I needed to nap most days. Although my clients gave me positive feedback about the therapy we did together, I felt that my brain was on hiatus sometimes due to the fatigue. I started to think about the things I wanted to do once I stopped working—taking piano lessons, reading more books, and spending time with friends that I hadn't before because of lack of energy.

By 2017, in all fairness to my clients and to myself, I decided I really needed to retire altogether in May of 2018. I began giving clients notice, so that they had time to make the adjustment and say goodbye, and I started providing recommendations for other therapists who could continue with them, if the client chose to continue therapy.

I have not regretted the decision to retire. Now that I don't have to push through each day, I am able to stimulate my brain—read a book or listen to a book or watch PBS or listen to NPR— and feel that I'm able to function. My life has been full with the exercise classes I attend, walking on a regular basis, napping almost daily, and still sleeping at least eight hours at night. Until COVID-19, I was playing mah-jongg a couple of times per month. I'm reading some of those books I accumulated through the years. I cook, and I have time to keep up with the news, although sometimes I don't want to. I play the piano daily and started taking piano lessons on Skype.

VI. DECIDING TO RETIRE

How do you know when you're ready to stop working?

I had been swimming against the current for quite some time, fighting the inevitable decisions that had to be made. I felt like a cliché— just another eighty-something, little old lady who didn't want to give up her independence, identity, home, lifestyle, or possessions. I kept talking about retirement as if it were some nebulous state of affairs that didn't apply to me. As I had said a hundred times, I didn't want to retire. I couldn't afford to retire; it just wasn't possible. On the other hand, I couldn't afford *not* to retire. This is what they call a Catch-22.

My three criteria for "closing my business" were (1) when there was no work, (2) when I couldn't do the work, or (3) when I no longer wanted to do the work. If even one of those options occurred, that's all it would take—just one—and I would retire.

1. When there was no work: I had clients who had signed letters of agreement and made down payments but then dropped off the radar. If they were doing any work on their books, I hadn't heard about it. I think I was more invested in their projects than they were.

2. When I couldn't do the work: I confess it was getting more difficult. This job takes patience, stamina, empathy, focus, and all the other traits I've written about for years, which I sensed were fading.

3. When I no longer wanted to do the work: That seemed to be where I was, feeling pretty burned out. I had earned a living as a writer for

fifty years and had been a successful entrepreneur for thirty of those years. It's possible that my last two difficult book projects took the starch out of me. I was tired, and I didn't want to do this anymore.

My three nonnegotiable criteria occurred simultaneously—a perfect storm that could not be rationalized away. For me, the decision to retire seemed straightforward, but I know this is not the way everyone decides to make this huge change in their lives. Having a choice about when you will stop working can make all the difference in how you view this major life transition. For example, if you have planned for your retirement, especially financially, and can afford to leave your job or your business, the timing is pretty much up to you. If you work for a company that has a mandatory retirement age, and you have reached it, the decision has been made for you. Sometimes, the state of your health may be the deciding factor. If your doctor tells you that you are putting your life at risk by continuing to work, the sensible decision is to stop.

That was what happened to my father. His doctor spelled out in plain language the consequences of continuing to work. Retiring was the last thing he wanted to do, but my father took his doctor's advice. He felt a bit lost for a while. I remember him asking me, "What does the man do when he doesn't work?" I thought for a long time that had more to do with his generation than his job. He had worked all his life. Our society is built on a strong work ethic, and leaving our work behind us is not always an easy transition.

I am very fortunate in that what I did for a living I can continue to do for the rest of my life, whether or not I get paid for it. Once you are a writer or an artist or involved in any creative activity, you never have to stop doing what you love. Writers write, and that is exactly what I intend to continue doing as long as I am able.

Asking the Tough Questions

Let's say none of these scenarios apply to you, and you are still struggling with whether to retire or keep working. Here are some questions you need to answer before you decide:

1. Can you afford to retire based on the money or investments you have?
A generally accepted rule of thumb for retirement planning is that for every year of retirement you should have at least 70 to 80 percent of the yearly salary you earned while you were working. According to *CNN Money*, "That might be enough *if* you've paid off your mortgage and are in excellent health when you kiss the office good-bye." But if you have big plans for your post-retirement years, you may need 100 percent or more of your annual income.

2. How much money will you need to live close to the lifestyle you're living now?
Take a hard look at your current expenses. Unless you cut them drastically, you're going to require at least what you are spending now. Add up all your sources of income— Social Security, savings accounts, investments, pension, 401k. If what you need is far more than what you have, consider postponing retirement for a while longer. If you have a financial advisor, by all means work with that person. In fact, that relationship should have begun long before you even thought about retirement.

3. How healthy are you and your spouse, if you have one?
Take an honest look at your health and how long you expect to live, barring unforeseen circumstances. If you are in excellent health and your family has longevity genes, you can keep working if you want to. On the other hand, if you or your spouse are in poor health, you probably don't want to postpone retiring. Then, if you can afford to, do as many of the things you were planning to do when you stopped working. Don't spend your time working when you could be living your life.

4. Do you and your spouse picture your retirement years in the same way?

This is something like planning a vacation. Your spouse thinks fishing for hours and cooking the catch over an open fire sounds like nirvana. You, on the other hand, prefer to be pampered and to dine in style. Imagine how different your images of retirement might be. Maybe you've been reading about retirement communities in Florida, while your other half is more inclined to just stay put in the home you've finally paid off. When you're married, you have to think of retirement as a team sport. You are in this together.

5. How much do you need to cover your healthcare now and in the foreseeable future?

It is no secret that the cost of healthcare in this country is rising beyond many people's ability to afford regular doctor visits, surgeries, or catastrophic events. Forty-four million people in this country have no health insurance today, and another thirty-eight million have inadequate coverage. If you are a sixty-five-year-old couple who is planning to retire in the near future, you will need between $200,000 and $400,000 to pay for healthcare. That is in addition to what Medicare already funds. To cover these costs, at the very least, you will need savings, private insurance, or a Medicare supplement policy.

6. Are you planning to live on your Social Security alone?

If you retire at sixty-two, your Social Security benefits would be 30 percent less than if you wait until your full retirement age. Early retirement reduces your benefits; retiring later increases them. Working until you are seventy results in maximum benefits. Retiring with no income other than Social Security may sound next to impossible. Yet, 23 percent of married retirees and 43 percent of single retirees count on their Social Security benefit for 90 percent or more of their monthly income. The question is how do they do it? Living mostly on Social Security alone can be difficult, but here are a few suggestions for how you can make it work.

» **First, be aware of the factors that will determine the amount of your benefits.** Once upon a time, sixty-five was considered normal retirement age, but that age has increased. Beginning with people born in 1938 or later, the age gradually increases until it reaches sixty-seven for people born after 1959. Assuming that Social Security is your only source of income, it's important to make this decision based on an honest assessment of your situation. If you are not in good health and don't believe you will live many years in retirement, you are probably better off applying for Social Security benefits sooner rather than later. Your monthly payment will be 76 percent higher if you wait until you are seventy, rather than applying for it at sixty-two. Staying in your job longer or finding part-time work will help you postpone taking your benefits early or permit you to live on the benefits you receive.

» **Do a Social Security do-over.** If you took Social Security early and now feel that was the wrong decision, you can change your mind. You have up to twelve months to withdraw your application and take advantage of the second-chance option. This Social Security do-over allows you to withdraw your application and then re-apply later if your financial situation unexpectedly changes. At that time, you must repay—without interest—all the benefits you received up to that point. But from then on, your benefit can grow until you're ready to file again. If the twelve-month deadline has passed, you have another chance to boost your benefit. Once you reach your full retirement age—currently sixty-six—you can suspend your monthly payments without having to repay the money you already received. Finally, you should be aware of survivor benefits. If you or your spouse dies, the survivor will receive whichever amount of Social Security is larger.

» **Eliminate debt.** This may seem obvious, but if you are in debt and planning to live mostly on Social Security when you retire, you're going to find it difficult, if not impossible, to make it work. Make a concerted effort to pay off your mortgage and as much high-interest-rate consumer debt, such as credit cards, as you can. If you still have credit-card debt when you retire, pay off as much as possible and cut up your credit cards so that you won't find yourself in that position again.

» **Move to a less expensive location.** Downsizing to a smaller place can lower your expenses, but if you want to maintain your present standard of living, consider moving somewhere with a lower cost-of-living where you can live on less money. *Bankrate*, a financial website, offers an online tool to compare living expenses from one place to another. For example, if your income is $50,000 a year in Boston, you would need only $30,942, or 38 percent less, to achieve the same standard of living in Augusta, Georgia.

» **Don't forget about taxes.** Don't let your tax bill catch you by surprise. Estimate what you think the taxes will be, and put that money aside every month. Before you choose a place to live when you retire, do some research. Not all states approach taxes in the same way. Fortunately, most of them, as well as the District of Columbia, don't tax Social Security benefits. Better yet, some states, such as Alaska, Florida, Nevada, South Dakota, Texas, Washington, and Wyoming, don't tax any income at all. Oregon and Delaware have no sales tax. Knowing these facts in advance could help you be more financially prepared.

» **Buddy up.** Think about getting a roommate or sharing your home with a friend. This is a good way to cut living expenses and prevent feeling isolated. According to the National Institute on

Aging (NIA), "As we age, many of us are alone more often than when we were younger, leaving us vulnerable to social isolation and loneliness—and related health problems such as cognitive decline, depression, and heart disease."

» **Be aware of helpful state and federal programs.** If you are struggling financially, you may qualify for one of these programs to help make ends meet. For example, "Extra Help" is designed to assist Medicare beneficiaries with limited income and resources to pay for prescription drugs. This assistance is estimated to be worth $4,000 a year for those enrolled in the Medicare prescription drug program. Find out more information on Extra Help, as well as other state and federal programs, at BenefitsCheckUp, a free service of the National Council on Aging (www.benefitscheckup.org).

» **Take advantage of free services.** Libraries, parks, and local museums offer a variety of free entertainment, including book reviews, free tours of art exhibits, concerts, and even Shakespeare in the park. Continuing-care retirement communities offer residents independent living, assisted living, and nursing-home care at different stages of their lives. Many of these communities open their programs and activities to the public, as well as to residents. If you have access to community colleges and universities, you can take advantage of their free lectures and other cultural programs. Most US schools allow older students to attend classes at no charge or at a significantly reduced rate. The best news is that, in this age of the Internet, you can take online courses at top universities or community colleges. Contrary to some of the commercials I've seen on TV, many of us are computer literate or have grandchildren who are only too happy to teach us anything we need to know about computers.

Obviously, there is more to the subject of retiring than I realized when I decided to do it. I confess I was not nearly as prepared as I should have been. There was so much I didn't know before I made the leap, and I suspect I was not alone. But one of the great advantages of being a writer is knowing how to find out anything you need to know. It's called research, and this book is the result of putting those skills to work to help all of us become better informed about retirement.

Larry Frost
Retired Teacher and Coach

Larry Frost was a high school teacher and coach for thirty-three years before he retired in 2010. He could have continued to work but decided it was time to spend more time with his family and do some of the things he hadn't been able to while he was working. Larry is an avid hunter who loves being out in nature with his sidekick, a beautiful chocolate lab named Cash. He also enjoys playing golf and spending time with his five grandchildren. Larry is currently on the board of the National Football Foundation (St. Louis Chapter), executive director of the St. Louis Metropolitan Football Coaches Association, and second vice president of the NFLPA Former Players (St. Louis Chapter). He also stays busy as a member of the Architectural and Building Committee in his community.

I taught school and coached at Clayton High School for twenty-eight years and then at Kirkwood for another six. (Clayton and Kirkwood are suburbs of St. Louis, Missouri.) I retired in 2010. There was no mandatory retirement age, so I could have continued to work. But I started thinking about time and family—my wife and children and grandchildren—and about some of the things I wanted to do but hadn't been able to because of my work schedule. I was ready to use my time the way I wanted to use it when I wanted to use it, rather than having to be someplace on somebody else's timetable.

I was at the point that what I was doing was no longer challenging. Coaching—getting players together, getting coaches together—seemed to fall into place more easily than it did before. And there were other things I wanted to do. When I put it all together, I knew it was time.

I wanted to play golf. It's not one of my favorite things to do, but I enjoy it. I really like to hunt. I like to get outdoors in the woods. That's mental therapy for me. And I wanted to spend time with my family. I have two grown children and five grandchildren—three boys and two girls.

I am doing some of those things now but not as much as I'd like. I'm having difficulty playing golf because of my joint pain. I'm not hunting as much as I want to, but I have gotten quite a bit in already this year. The pandemic hasn't stopped me from hunting, but it has stopped me from hunting with some of the people I like to hunt with. I do get out in the woods for turkey hunting, but as far as getting in close quarters for duck hunting, that's not possible right now. If this were duck season, we would still be able to hunt, but we would probably be some distance apart, which would mean two people instead of three. If we were out on a boat fishing, we would be in some pretty close quarters. These are some things we will have to work through. The big thing is that, because COVID-19 can be asymptomatic, people who don't even know they have it could be passing it along. *I* could be passing it along. Who knows?

The kids were the best part about teaching. They kept me young. That's the part I miss, as well as well as competing against other coaches. The most difficult part, as I got older and advanced in my career, was that the parents and paperwork and bureaucracy were taking more time, and I couldn't do some of the things I used to do that were beneficial to the kids.

Kids definitely need limits and boundaries, and as I stayed in teaching longer, I wasn't seeing that as much in the youngsters because they weren't getting it at home. I think this does kids a disservice because as they get older, if they haven't had boundaries and limits, suddenly having them can be traumatic. It's a matter of letting kids know that they are responsible for their actions.

This is probably not their fault. If you look at kids in grade school and middle school, they haven't had to fend for themselves. When I was raising my kids, I wanted to make sure that, when they got to a certain point, they could do whatever they needed to do on their own. Back then, I felt that we had done our job raising them. Today, often, that is not the case. It's more like parents don't want to hurt their kids' feelings. They want to be friends.

When I was growing up, the boundaries I had were related to having respect for people who were older and more experienced. The most important thing I learned was that you should never embarrass your mom and dad. That was instilled in us. Today, if you have holes in your jeans, that's the style. But then, if we had a hole in our jeans or our shirt, we couldn't wear those things until they were sewn because we didn't want people to think we were poor.

Our parents grew up in the Depression era. When I was barely able to walk, I remember little things like, if we left the room and we didn't turn out the lights, we were in trouble. And water... we didn't flush the toilet every time we used it, and baths and showers were quick. Everything was at a premium. You couldn't just use something; you had to make sure you used it wisely.

During this pandemic, many people are doing a balancing act between their livelihood and their well-being. A lot of people with young families are asking, *What am I going to do?* I keep thinking about all of those people who are not working and need those stimulus checks—the people with small businesses and those who are not working right now. This is tough. Until they come up with something where they can say, okay, we can treat this virus, and you're going to be okay, we are really going to have to change the way we live.

It isn't easy to live on Social Security for those who have nothing else. First of all, they don't give you much, and they have taken and borrowed from it for so long that there's practically nothing there. As a former teacher, my retirement plan is outstanding. When I was teaching, I put in 12 percent of my salary; now, I think it's up to 16 percent. It all goes toward retirement. So, you do without while you're working, but you make up for it later. In Missouri, the retirement system for teachers is excellent.

A lot of men—more men than women, I think—just don't know how to stop working. They ask, *What am I going to do with myself?* I'm not one of those people. When I retired, I wanted to retire. I felt good about it. I figured that I would get a certain amount of money, and it was actually more than I was getting when I was working. I also had savings—not a great deal but enough to invest in something—and my medical was paid for when I reached sixty-five. At that point, my kids were both out of the house and married and on their own. So I was pretty well set.

Now I spend more time with my wife. When I was working, we hardly went out—but since I retired, we've been able to do that a little more than before. We've done some traveling, such as going on a couple of cruises. We were planning to go to Alaska in June, but the pandemic canceled that trip.

I never had a bucket list; if I did, it was a pretty small bucket. I don't think I had expectations about retirement, but the feeling of knowing that I was definitely free, that I didn't have to go someplace and work, was probably the best feeling I've had. Knowing I didn't have to be accountable to someone or something all the time was wonderful.

Retirement to me is a blessing—to not have to account for my time. The number one thing, right now, is time. For a while I guess I thought I was never going to die, but now I know it's going to happen. I spend a lot of time thinking about it and the fact that we don't really have a choice about when, where, or how it's going to happen. It just will. I think about how I want it, where I want it—all that. I know that I'm just a visitor here, and that sooner or later, my time is going to be up.

Andi and Pete Krehbiel
On Moving to a Retirement Community

Andi and Pete grew up in Chicago and started their careers in education after college. After heading counseling departments in Illinois and Arizona, Pete went into private practice as a psychotherapist. Andi taught school and held various positions in education in Illinois and Arizona before becoming an advocate for families with special-needs children. Both have advanced degrees—Andi in education and Pete in counseling—and have been adjunct instructors in master's programs at several universities.

Andi

Part of why we decided to move into a retirement community when we had a house was because the house was twenty-five years old, and it was starting to require some work. We had never had the roof repaired, which was probably the next thing on the list. And then the air conditioning was beginning to go. The more we talked about it, the more we saw that repairing a house that we were probably not going to be in for another twenty-five years was not the way we wanted to spend our money.

If we decided to fix things, we would need help. Pete's health is not such that he is able to do a lot of the things that would have to be done, like climbing on ladders and changing twelve-foot-ceiling lightbulbs. He didn't want to take care of the yard, and I don't blame him. I don't want to take care of the yard either. We knew the situation wasn't going to get any better. We didn't want to keep having to ask our children to come over and do things for us, and we didn't want to spend money to hire repair people all the time or have someone come out just to change the lightbulbs.

We did a lot of research before we chose this place. We started our planning by going to a facility that wasn't going to be ready for four years. We were thinking of moving there with other friends of ours. We all went to look at it, and we all liked it. But the more we looked into it, the more we found that it was not going to use green construction materials. We decided to keep looking. Since we had already started on this journey, we went to a bunch of other places. I knew the place we live in now because I used to take classes here. We know this is not for everybody, but for us, this was a good choice because it doesn't have a continuum of care all the way through nursing care. Therefore, it is less expensive.

We talked to our lawyer; we talked to our financial planners; we talked to people we knew; and we came here several times. They all said the same thing. Their first question was do you have long-term health insurance? And we do. We've had it for years, so they told us we didn't need to go to a place that has a continuum of care. This is a good thing because anywhere you go that has continuing care, you have to buy into it. It is over $1 million to buy in, and we didn't have that kind of money.

We asked our financial planners if we had enough money to move in and live here for a while. After all, we don't know how old we are going to be or how long we're going to live. They figured out with our resources how much we would have to spend each year if we were living in the way that we wanted to live, and they said, "Yes, you have enough money. Go ahead and do it, and do it now. Don't wait till you're too old to enjoy the life this senior retirement community can provide for you."

That's why we did it. I was thrilled to death; Pete, not so much. His whole reaction to all of this was, "I'm not ready, but you keep insisting, so we'll do it." But the truth is, we didn't want to believe we're as old as we are. Once we came to terms with the fact that, yes, we are this old, and, yes, it's progressive and will get more complicated, not less, it was another factor in helping us decide.

I had health issues that were resolved, but I think I was scared too. I don't know where these things came from; I don't know what's going to come next; and I was worried about Pete being left alone. We have four kids. Two of them live here; one of them is moving away. We thought, *Where are we going to go?* If we follow our children, they may not stay where they are, so which one do you pick? We just decided we were going to do this for ourselves.

I'm thrilled that I did it. I was happy the first weekend we were here. It's everything I wanted it to be. The only thing I don't like about it is that the older people I like very much keep getting sick or dying, but other than that, I love it. I sold my car. First of all, we don't go to many places where we need a car anymore, and if I really need a car, they have that service here. If I need to go to the doctor or something like that, we try to figure out a good plan where both of us could use Pete's car on different days and make our appointments that way. Having just one car has been a learning experience for us, but when I want to see my friends, I just sign up and book a ride.

Pete said he was never going to "get involved," that he didn't want any part of anything. But in the meantime, he plays pool with four other guys every week, and he has become really involved in painting. He's in the art studio a lot. The facility gives scholarships to the kids who work here to go to college and paint. Pete is on the scholarship committee. So, even though he said, "No, I'm never going to do anything," he's doing quite a bit.

When we moved in here, we met a lot of people who said, "Well, this is our last home. This is the end of the road." Pete and I don't feel that way. We don't know if this is our last home because we don't know what life is going to bring us. It's not a question of age; it's just a question of the uncertainty.

Pete

I was not as gung-ho on doing this as Andi was, although we had looked at other places with some friends of ours who were thinking about it, too. What's good for one person is not necessarily good for others, and the friends we started out with on this journey did not come here. They moved somewhere else, so that's just how it is.

I'll tell you what I like. I like the community. I like a lot of the people. I've made some good friends here. What I don't like is being significantly younger than many of them and watching them go through the progression of deterioration. Andi said something similar—that it's so hard for her to watch people get sick or die. And we see a lot of that.

I like being able to help people. I helped someone this morning who was trying to sell her car. I met with her and this gentleman who wanted to buy it. I'm on a scholarship committee with the kids who work here, and I like that part. The part I don't like is watching people age in front of me, and of course I know I'm aging at the same time. But I'm seeing a lot of dementia, maybe more than some of the other people here can see it. I can pick up on this because I was a licensed professional counselor in private practice for twenty years or more.

I *am* kicking and screaming about aging. I keep wondering if anybody really comes to grips with getting old. Maybe some do it better than others. I've had days where I feel like I am young again, and then I have other days where I feel physically old.

VII. TALKING TO YOUR (ADULT) CHILDREN

Can you (and they) face the tough questions?

REMEMBER WHEN YOU WERE the undisputed authority in your home, and your children didn't question your role as a parent? Remember when you could say, "You are grounded," or, "No, you can't sleep at Bobby's tonight," or, "Yes, you can use the car, but be home before eleven." If that seems like a long time ago, it probably was. You are a little (well, a lot) older now, and your children aren't children anymore. It seems like overnight they became adults, and your role as the authority in your family has flipped on its head.

Do we really need all that help? And if so, when? There is no magic age when we are considered old and in need of constant monitoring and care. Our kids may be stressed out over feeling obligated to help us, but it is equally stressful for us to find ourselves the recipients of help we don't think we need and to feel our independence slipping away.

It happens in small ways. They accompany us to doctor visits and often talk to the doctor as if we aren't even there. They check to see if we have eaten or taken our meds when we are perfectly capable of doing both. They monitor the "sell-by" date on food in the refrigerator and immediately assume we have dementia.

And so, bit by bit, we lose our independence, especially when we begin to find it difficult to take care of ourselves or manage our own lives.

For example, a loss of mobility is frustrating simply because we can't get around as well as we once did. When we have difficulty climbing the stairs, walking short distances without assistance, standing up, or getting out of bed—all things we used to be able to do for ourselves—these become both a logistical issue and a blow to our self-image. Memory loss, vision or hearing problems, or even reduced stamina can affect our ability to live alone, drive, prepare meals, keep a house clean, and more. The loss of a spouse can also put us in a position where independent living may become more difficult and less safe.

Of course, not all of us react the same way about our loss of independence. Responses may range from anger and frustration to feelings of vulnerability and helplessness. We may be sad or afraid or confused. When we can no longer live on our own, many of us struggle with the loss of our homes, our possessions, our health, our body parts, and our vocations, not to mention our independence. Explaining to our adult children why these issues are so important to us is not always easy, especially if they feel that we need their help.

Being independent means you will be able to go through challenging life situations, as you always have, without always depending on your children to help you cope. You will be able to pay your own bills and control your income and expenditures. You will be more comfortable making decisions without having to wonder how your children will react. You will have freedom to explore your skills and talents and be prepared to meet new people and try new things. Finally, and perhaps most important, the *more independent you are, the greater your self-confidence and self-esteem will be.*

Another difficult subject, especially for your adult children, is the need to put your affairs in order before the end of your life. You may be quite comfortable talking about what has to be done, how you want to be cared for, and your preferences regarding your funeral; but believe me, your children may not be as open to this conversation as you are.

You have had plenty of time to contemplate the whole subject of dying; your children, no matter how old they are, would prefer to think you are immortal. I experienced this when my own mother was dying (in her nineties) and when I bring up the subject to one of my daughters.

Yes, it's a painful subject but one that must be addressed. If no one does it, your friends and family members will have no idea what you really want. I know this is an extreme example, but I remember well the Terry Schiavo case. Her parents fought to keep her alive, even though she was in a persistent vegetative state, but her husband insisted that she would not have wanted to live this way. If Ms. Schiavo's desires had been expressed in the legally prescribed way, perhaps this argument, which garnered national attention in the press, could have been prevented.

While people are living longer, most of us will deal with some chronic condition or disability. The goal is to live with as much control and quality of life as possible, and that quality of life should extend to the very end. To ensure that it does, you need to have several important documents for end-of-life planning: a will, advance directives, a durable power of attorney for healthcare decisions, and funeral and burial/cremation preferences. It is better to have these documents in place *before* you are diagnosed with a life-threatening illness, when the need suddenly becomes urgent.

In the midst of coping with the medical, emotional, psychological, and spiritual challenges of having a serious illness, you or your children will also have to manage mundane logistical details. If you don't address them now, someone—probably your children—will have to address them later.

Making a Will
More than half of adults in this country don't have a will. But you need one, even if you don't have a vast estate to distribute among your heirs. People who die without a will send their loved ones to court to navigate

the probate process and to deal with dividing up property while they're still grieving. The question is this: Do you want to determine where your assets go, or do you want the state to do it?

Writing a will isn't that difficult. There are a number of inexpensive online will-writing programs, although hiring a family-law attorney to draft one is a better alternative. The costs vary depending on where you live and how complicated your situation is, but you will be glad you invested in having a will prepared correctly. In addition to stipulating where you want your property to go, your will or accompanying documents should also include papers outlining your plans for guardianship of minor children, if you have any.

Advance Directives

Sometimes called a living will, this document spells out the measures you would like taken, or not taken, to prolong your life. Living wills and other advance directives are legal instructions regarding your preferences for medical care if you are unable to make decisions for yourself. Advance directives guide choices for doctors and caregivers if you are terminally ill, seriously injured, in a coma, in the late stages of dementia, or near the end of life. Even the healthiest person could experience a sudden accident and not be able to speak for herself. But when you have a life-threatening illness, it's particularly important to make clear, in writing, what your wishes are in case you can't express them yourself.

By planning ahead, you can get the medical care you want, avoid unnecessary suffering, and relieve family members of the need to make decisions during moments of crisis or grief. You also help reduce confusion or disagreement about the choices you would want people to make on your behalf.

Durable Power of Attorney for Healthcare

Designating someone to have your power of attorney for healthcare does not mean you give up any power to make your own decisions.

But there may come a point when you cannot speak for yourself. At that point, you will need someone to make decisions for you, such as whether or not you would want to be kept alive on a ventilator. This person should have a copy of your advance directives and should know your specific wishes regarding the kinds of lifesaving measures you do and do not want.

Instructions for Your Funeral or Memorial Service
When someone has just died, grieving family members must often think quickly about plans for funerals or memorial services. Immediately following a death, it can be hard to focus on details, such as what your favorite song was or what kind of burial you would prefer. Sit down with someone you trust—preferably one of your adult children—to brainstorm about necessary details. Then, write down all the things that are important to you about your funeral, memorial service, and how your body is to be dealt with. Here are some questions to think about:

- Do you want a funeral or memorial service? In a church, synagogue, mosque, or somewhere else? Who should preside?
- What would you like to have read, sung, or said at your service? Is there someone you would like to have speak?
- Would you like your body to be viewed after your death? By close family only?
- Would you like to record an audio or video message for a service after your death?
- How would you like your body to be dealt with? Do you prefer burial or cremation?
- How do you feel about organ donation or donating your body to medical research?

A Palliative Care Team Can Help
A palliative care team, usually recommended by your primary care physician, can help you find a financial planner, attorney, or other

professionals who can ensure that your wishes are carried out and respected. In general, the interdisciplinary palliative care team includes a doctor, a nurse, and a social worker; but other experts often fill out the team according to a patient's needs. These can include chaplains, counselors, pharmacists, dietitians, habilitation specialists, physical therapists, music and art therapists, and home-health aides. Your palliative care team can provide the following services:

- Relieve pain and other symptoms
- Address your emotional and spiritual concerns, as well as your family's
- Coordinate your care
- Improve your quality of life during your illness
- Help your family by offering medical information, emotional support, and home-care assistance

The subject of your death can be hard for your children to talk about calmly and rationally. It might be difficult for you, as well, if you have not come to terms with your own mortality. So your approach to the subject and your efforts to take your children's feelings into account will make all the difference in how the conversation goes. When my parents were older, I lived in a different city. Once, when I came to visit them, my father took me to their safe deposit box and showed me the contents so I would know what preparations they had made. Not the most pleasant afternoon I ever spent, but it did relieve many of my concerns.

Sometimes you don't have an earthshaking topic to discuss and yet still find it difficult to talk to your children. Perhaps your relationship is not all that it could be, or either you or your children need to brush up on your communication skills. Whatever the reason, at this stage of the game, changing years of ingrained patterns might be not be easy. But even if the conversation is small talk or lighthearted banter, it is worth a try.

My mother and I didn't always have smooth communication, but the most amazing thing happened when she turned eighty. We could talk to each other. Perhaps we had both changed, but whatever happened was a gift that lasted for twelve years. I always wished this gift had arrived earlier, but I treasured the time we did have talking and laughing and enjoying each other. So if things aren't exactly as you would like them to be right now, don't lose heart. They could change when you least expect them to.

Joann Dyroff
Attorney at Law

Joann Dyroff is an experienced personal and business attorney with a diverse practice, including estate planning, probate and trust administration, business planning, entity creation and oversight, tax, charitable and nonprofit organizations, and pension and profit-sharing plans, including division of those plans in divorce. A primary focus of her practice is on consultation with individuals regarding estate-planning matters, preparation of estate-planning documents on behalf of individuals and families, and trust and probate administration. Ms. Dyroff works with a number of nonprofit organizations providing guidance on incorporation, as well as operational and management issues.

◆ ◆ ◆

What Documents Do You Need?
There are certain documents that everyone should have that are used during that person's lifetime.

A Durable Power of Attorney for financial matters allows someone to handle your financial matters in the event you can no longer act for yourself, e.g., to pay bills, file tax returns, and handle other day-to-day documents on your behalf.

A Healthcare Declaration and Durable Power of Attorney for Healthcare allows you to state your intention of what you would or wouldn't want to have done if you are incapacitated and perhaps in a vegetative state. Sometimes this is also called a living will. It also names someone to make healthcare decisions for you if you are unable to speak for yourself.

Sometimes these forms are available on a state website, such as the Missouri Bar. Another form for a healthcare declaration is a document available online called "The Five Wishes," which has both a living will and the power of attorney for healthcare and is legal in most states.

Everyone needs to have those documents in place to handle financial and medical issues in the event of physical or mental disability. If these documents are not in place, there may be a need for a court guardianship or conservatorship, which means that the court has to determine if you are incompetent and, if so, appoint someone to act for you. It can be a difficult and expensive process for a family to have doctors assert and a court rule that you are incompetent and then have someone appointed who is required to continually report to the court. Having a power of attorney for financial and healthcare matters can avoid the need for a guardianship/conservatorship proceeding in probate court.

A HIPAA Release Authorization names people who can talk to your doctors in the hospital or other medical providers but doesn't authorize those individuals to make decisions on your behalf.

These documents are effective during your lifetime. Following your death, documents, such as a Last Will and Testament and a trust can be critical.

How Should You Pass Along Your Assets?
Once death occurs, your assets will pass as you determine under your will or a trust, or as provided under state law.

The probate process is required if you have assets in your name alone at the time of your death, and a court will use your Last Will and Testament to determine where the assets should pass at your death. A will normally also names the person whom you wish to handle your estate and waives the requirement for a bond. If you don't have a will in place, the court will ensure that your assets are transferred as provided under state law. In addition, the person who is appointed to handle your probate estate is determined under state law, and a bond may be required before that person can be appointed.

You can avoid probate if you hold your assets in joint names or have a beneficiary designation for your assets, because those assets will pass to the joint owner or to the named beneficiary. However, even if all of your assets are held in joint names with a spouse or child, if that individual predeceases you, the asset may need to pass through probate. If a husband and wife have assets together and the wife dies first, unless some other action has been taken, those assets are now in the husband's name, and they may have to be transferred through the probate process with court involvement.

Another way to avoid probate is to create a revocable trust during your lifetime and to have your assets owned by the trust or pass to your trust at the time of death under a beneficiary designation. The trust does not die; your named successor becomes the trustee upon your death or disability, and assets held by the trust can avoid probate.

Family issues can often complicate the situation following death. Mark Twain once said that you don't really know someone until you have shared an inheritance with them. Family members can disagree over personal property or household items, as well as over division of investments and real estate. They can get really upset about what happened to the old Christmas ornaments or Mom's rings or the Hummel collection. Those things may not have great monetary value, but often those personal, sentimental items become very important to family members.

Do You Need an Attorney?

I recommend having an attorney to prepare these documents. Some of the powers of attorney and healthcare forms are available from state bar associations and other websites, and those may work well for some.

Wills and trusts are more complicated documents. While you can look at legal websites and create basic documents, there may be words and phrases in those documents that you don't really understand but that can have important ramifications. The documents may not allow you to think through important issues, such as when should your children receive property or what happens if your primary beneficiaries are not living at the time of your death. The problem is that you don't know what you don't know. That makes it more dangerous to use and entirely depend on those documents.

It is important to have all these documents in place and to talk with family members about your wishes. This is an emotional subject, and at the time of disability or death, family members may react in unexpected ways. It's a good idea to think things through and make your wishes known while you are able to.

Do You Need a DNR?

A DNR (Do Not Resuscitate) is a form typically used in a hospital or nursing home and is not part of a standard healthcare declaration. Someone acting under a medical power of attorney may have the authority to complete a DNR for a patient.

Some states also allow an "Out of Hospital DNR" to be signed, but in most states, this also requires a doctor to sign the form. A DNR is for very limited circumstances. You need to understand what it does and when you need one. The DNR normally provides that, if you are in the hospital or a nursing home, you would not want to be resuscitated in the event of a heart attack or other serious medical emergency. My concern is whether a DNR form allows some discretion to be used if, for example, you are in an accident that you could recover from with some extra medical intervention and live another twenty years. A case in Florida several years ago involved a man who was brought into the emergency room, and he had "Do Not Resuscitate" tattooed on his chest. He could have survived his medical emergency with no long-term consequences had he been treated, but the hospital was unable to reach any family members and only had the directions he had provided via his tattoo. He was not treated, and he died.

My personal view is that a DNR is for limited circumstances, such as someone who is suffering from a terminal disease. If he is not going to get better, and he knows he is not going to survive except in a vegetative state or subject to great pain, and he doesn't want extraordinary methods taken to keep him alive, a DNR may be appropriate. Or, if the patient has severe dementia and has made it clear to her family that she wouldn't want to live this way, a DNR may be appropriate.

A person living at home who believes strongly that he would not want to be resuscitated in the event of a medical emergency needs to make it clear to his family not to call 911 in the event of such an emergency. If someone calls 911, the paramedics are going to come, and they may be required to try to resuscitate him.

Eileen Carlson
Willing to Confront Tough Topics

My husband, Clare, and I just redid our will about a month ago because circumstances and situations change and because you should do it every few years. My parents were older when they wrote their will. My brother, Sheldon, and I were there. My son, Mark, lived in Southern California, near my parents, so he was there, too. We were talking about the will, and Mark and Sheldon asked more questions than I did. I just listened. Mark said to my dad, "I don't think what you're doing is fair, Grandpa, because you're leaving a lot of money to me because of the grandkids. That's not fair to the rest of the family." So, my dad changed it and left the bulk of the estate to Sheldon and me and some to the grandchildren as well.

My mother was not terribly involved in the conversation. My dad was a businessman, and I think the best solution is to be able to talk about things from a business perspective and work them out in the way that's best for all the parties concerned. I think that's what he was doing.

Clare and I had that same conversation recently, and we felt that we had to change our will. One reason was that we were living in a different state than where the will was originally written. So, we went to a lawyer, and we revised our documents. When we talked to our daughter, Robyn, she had some concerns.

Our son had borrowed some money from us, and Robyn didn't think it was right that he was not paying it back. He had asked us to take out a mortgage on our house in Colorado, which was paid off, so he could buy a piece of a business. We did take out the mortgage, and he did buy into the business. It was a loan he was supposed to pay back. He had not done so yet. When we went to our accountant, he told us, "You're paying way more money than you need to. Either forgive the interest or forgive the loan." We chose to forgive the interest and left the loan in place.

When we divided up the money we would leave our kids, we subtracted the amount Mark borrowed. We told him we were doing that. We have a really good relationship with our grandchildren, so the other thing we did was to give some money to each of them. Robyn has no problem with that at all. She has no problem with Mark getting a share and his children getting a share and Clare's daughter, Kristin, getting a share. For all of us, the issue is *fairness*.

What's easy is, now that they're grown up, they don't mind talking about this subject. When we got together, the meeting was between the Robins (Robyn's husband is also named Robin) and Clare and me. Mark is happy with whatever we do because we loaned him the money. After that point, nothing happened until we sold the house, and we got less money than we would have gotten without the mortgage. That was not a surprise.

I think it's significant that when the Robins recently picked up some stuff for us and brought it over, they wouldn't come near us. We stood on the deck, and they stood on the bulkhead. Robyn said, "I couldn't stand it if by some strange quirk of fate, we would bring the coronavirus, and you would get sick and die. I just couldn't stand that." So, their concern is primarily that we live as long as we can as well as we can, and we'll worry about the other stuff later. That has been my experience with my daughter.

But the upshot is that we are all able to talk to each other, and if people have concerns, we can talk them out. It's kind of unusual. I had no trepidation about bringing the subject up with my kids or with my parents. Fortunately, both of my parents were cognizant of everything until the day they died. My mother died at ninety-four, and two days before she died, she said, "Well, at least I still have my marbles." They were both still smart at the end, and that's a gift.

I haven't thought a lot about death until the last three months when it has been on my mind because of the medical diagnosis I received recently. I had to face reality. I don't know if that's why we chose to do the will again, but you have to face your mortality. That's not easy in our society. We don't talk about dying.

My advice to parents of all ages: I think the most important thing is to make sure your lines of communication are open and you can talk to one another.

VIII. FIGURING OUT YOUR FINANCES

Are you prepared to retire?

THE ONE SUBJECT NO SENIOR CITIZEN can afford to ignore is also the one subject many of us find uncomfortable to discuss: Money. There seem to be two extremes: At one end of the spectrum are those who have thought through and planned every aspect of their retirement; at the other end are those who are retiring on a wing and prayer, with little to no planning and limited financial resources. For this group, the subject is particularly tough. Not only are they unprepared, often they don't know what they don't know.

At any time of one's life, money can be a confusing and emotional topic. When money is tight and today's bills are piling up, preparing for retirement isn't even on the radar. Of course, it's better to start thinking about saving and investing while you're still young, but like so many people, you may find yourself staring at the end of your work life before you were even prepared to think about your financial situation.

The touchstone for any discussion of aging and finances seems to be the 76.4 million Baby Boomers, who were born between 1946 and 1964. By 2030, all 76-plus million of them will be sixty-five or older. In the meantime, according to the *Washington Post,* "Each day, 10,000 Baby Boomers retire and begin receiving Medicare and Social Security benefits." Unfortunately, "The vast majority will not have sufficient savings to retire full-time at sixty-five with their pre-retirement standard of living."

That's one of the sobering conclusions from the recent *Sightlines* report issued by the Stanford Center on Longevity (SCL).

As a result, if you are approaching retirement, you will either need to work beyond age sixty-five, reduce your standard of living, or do some combination of the two. Wrapping your head around your financial future may seem daunting, but what follows are the basic building blocks. You can tap into any of these sources for funds except long-term healthcare. They include Social Security, investments in later life, wills and estate planning, and creating a paycheck during your retirement. (O'Neill, *Financial Fitness for the Rest of Your Life*)

SOCIAL SECURITY

Many of us over sixty-five have come to depend on Social Security, which is the largest source of income most of us have. Full retirement age (FRA) for anyone born in 1937 or before is sixty-five. You can retire early, at sixty-two, if you wish, but your benefits will be lower than if you wait.

What You Need to Know

You must have paid Social Security taxes for at least ten years before you apply. The good news is, if you wait until you reach your FRA, you can continue to work as long as you wish and earn as much as you can without reducing your benefit. If you apply early (at sixty-two), your benefits will be permanently reduced, and there may be a limit to what you can earn. The next part is somewhat confusing. To claim your full benefit, you need to sign up for Social Security at your full retirement age, *which varies by birth year.*

If you think sixty-five is still the age when everyone can apply for Social Security, you are incorrect. The FRA is sixty-five for those born in 1937 or earlier. For every year beyond 1937 up to 1943, add two months to your birthday month. If you were born between 1943 and

1954, your FRA will be sixty-six. Then, the system goes back to adding two months to your birthday. If you were born in 1970 or later, you can start collecting Social Security at sixty-seven.

| Age to Receive Full Social Security Benefits ||
YEAR OF BIRTH*	FULL RETIREMENT AGE
1937 or earlier	65
1938	65 and 2 months
1939	65 and 4 months
1940	65 and 6 months
1941	65 and 8 months
1942	65 and 10 months
1943–1954	66
1955	66 and 2 months
1956	66 and 4 months
1957	66 and 6 months
1958	66 and 8 months
1959	66 and 10 months
1960 and later	67

If you were born on January 1st of any year, you should refer to the previous year. (If you were born on the 1st of the month, your benefit and your full retirement age is figured as if your birthday was in the previous month.)

The earliest you can start receiving Social Security retirement benefits will remain age sixty-two. If you delay your retirement benefits until FRA, you also may be eligible for delayed retirement credits that would increase your monthly benefit. If you decide to delay your retirement, be sure to **sign up for Medicare at age sixty-five.**

After you begin collecting Social Security, you will receive a Social Security Earnings and Benefit Estimate Statement every year. Always check that statement to be sure it is correct. If it isn't, call Social Security at 1-800-772-1213.

Don't wait until your sixty-fifth birthday to put the wheels in motion. Contact Social Security about three months before your sixty-fifth birthday to make an appointment. You will be required to bring your Social Security card, birth certificate, proof of citizenship (if you were not born in the United States); your spouse's birth certificate, Social Security number, and marriage certificate (if you are married); military discharge papers (if you have been in the service); and your most recent W-2 form or tax return (if you are self-employed).

Social Security certainly makes life easier for many people, but it doesn't always provide enough to maintain your present lifestyle. If you have figured out how much you will need to live when you retire, calculate the difference between that amount and how much you will receive in Social Security benefits. Then, decide how you are going to cover the gap between those two numbers. Many older adults who thought they could live on Social Security are realizing that they will need to supplement their benefit. However, if you are getting divorced, and you were married at least ten years and don't remarry, you can qualify for benefits based on your ex-spouse's earnings when you both reach age sixty-two. You will receive whichever is higher—benefits based on your own work history or half of your ex-spouse's benefit.

HEALTH AND LONG-TERM CARE INSURANCE

The rule of thumb is that unless you are covered by your employer until you are eligible for Medicare, you should consider buying health insurance to tide you over until your FRA. It's wise to supplement your Medicare with long-term care insurance because all it takes is one surgery or serious illness to wipe out all of your savings. About half of all personal bankruptcies are the result of unpaid medical bills.

What You Need to Know

Medicare covers people age sixty-five and over, those under sixty-five with disabilities, and people of all ages with permanent kidney failure.

But in many cases, it only covers 80 percent of your medical costs. If you don't want to pay that amount out of pocket, be prepared to buy a supplemental or Medigap policy, which pays expenses that Medicare doesn't cover. While it's an additional monthly bill, I can attest to its value. If you have to pay for what Medicare doesn't cover after a surgery or an unexpected hospitalization, you will wish you had bought a Medigap policy.

Medigap policies are provided by private insurance companies, and their costs vary greatly, so it pays to do your homework. COBRA health insurance allows you to keep your existing health insurance so you stay protected. (COBRA stands for Consolidated Omnibus Budget Reconciliation Act. It was passed by Congress in 1985 as a way for people to continue health insurance coverage for a period of time after losing group coverage due to leaving a job.) COBRA can be a "stopgap" measure until you have health insurance covered by a new employer or Medicare.

Medicare can be confusing, especially with commercials on television urging you to buy a Part C Medicare Advantage plan instead of Parts A, B, and D. To clear up any confusion, coverage consists of the following:

- **Part A** covers hospital care, including emergency care, home health, long-term help, and hospice. You can enroll in part A when you are first eligible for Medicare.
- **Part B** covers doctor's visits, preventive care, outpatient procedures, medical equipment, labs, and dialysis. If you don't get part B when you are first eligible, your monthly premium may go up 10 percent for each twelve-month period. In most cases, you'll have to pay this late-enrollment penalty each time you pay for your premiums, and the penalty increases the longer you go without Part B coverage.
- **Part C** (Medicare Advantage) provides hospital and medical coverage through a managed-care plan (e.g., HMOs and PPOs). Medicare contracts with insurance carriers to offer Medicare part C; be sure you understand what part C covers before you sign up.

- **Part D** is a voluntary, outpatient prescription drug benefit offered by private insurance plans.

Long-term care, which is not covered by Medicare, covers a wide range of services from assistance at home with daily activities to care in a nursing home. Don't wait until you need it to buy long-term health insurance. You'll probably be in better health, and the cost will be lower if you buy it when you are fifty-five to sixty. The key is to find a balance between the coverage you want and the premium you can afford. As you look at long-term care coverage, be sure you understand how much it pays per day, how long the coverage lasts, exactly what is covered, and how long you have to wait to receive your benefits. All of these factors affect the price of the policy.

What You Need to Do
Apply for Medicare within three months of your sixty-fifth birthday (or the birthday at which you are eligible). If you are still working, contact your employer's Human Resources Department, and ask how your organization's health insurance or COBRA benefits interacts with Medicare. Contact your local State Health Insurance Assistance Program (SHIP) office or a financial advisor to help you choose the best Medigap and long-term care insurance for you. If you look up SHIP online, it is difficult to sort through all the offerings and links, so guidance from a financial advisor or an insurance agent you trust is a better way to choose the right policies.

If your family is helping to pay for your long-term health insurance, explain to them what long-term health insurance covers and how much it costs. Go over the details of the plan or ask your insurance agent to walk them through the policy.

Every day, we hear about people who have experienced identity theft and health-insurance fraud. Everyone is vulnerable, which I found out when someone applied for my IRS refund using all my information. I was not alone in being a victim of that particular scam. Protect your personal information and Medicare and Social Security numbers, and shred all healthcare documents before your throw them out.

LATER-LIFE INVESTMENT DECISIONS

If you are thinking about investing in your later years, expect to receive conflicting advice from friends and family. Some may advise you to invest more conservatively than you did when you were younger (i.e., hold less stock and more bonds and cash assets); others will warn that your investments have to last a long time—perhaps into your 70s, 80s, and 90s—so you should be a bit more aggressive and look at stocks, rather than bonds. While stocks have provided the highest return over time, investing in them has its risks, especially if share prices decline.

What You Need to Know

Let's say that, up to this point, you have been saving as much as you can and planning for the future. Here are some suggestions for ways to make your savings grow: Put away as much money as you possibly can. Ask your employer how much you can contribute to your 401k or any other tax-deferred plan your company provides. The maximum annual contribution for traditional and/or Roth individual retirement accounts (IRAs) was $6,000 in 2019, plus an additional catch-up contribution of up to $1,000 for people who are fifty or older and are still earning income. If possible, fund your employer's tax-deferred plan up to the maximum—usually 6 percent of your salary.

How do you decide where to put your money? According to The New Jersey Coalition for Financial Education (NJCFE), to provide $1,000 of monthly income in retirement, you will need to set aside approximately $300,000. Second, where you will invest depends on how much risk you can tolerate. Just as some of your advisors told you, stocks and mutual funds have historically earned two to three times the yield on bonds. One way to avoid a significant loss is with a diversified portfolio of stocks, bonds, and cash assets.

Tax-deferred plans, such as IRAs and 401ks, are not investment products; they are "umbrella" accounts into which specific investments are placed. Retirement plans with your employer's matching funds means your contribution is essentially "free money," so it makes sense to sign up for one when you first begin working. Rollovers of funds from one tax-deferred retirement savings plan to another must be completed within sixty days of the date of distribution of funds.

What You Need to Do

Investing at any age is complicated unless you are an expert. If you are not, it's wise to hire a professional advisor to guide you through the process. To find an advisor, visit these websites:

- Financial Planning Association (fpanet.org)
- National Association of Personal Financial Advisors (napfa.org)
- Certified Financial Planner Board of Standards (cfp-board.org)

Take advantage of all available investment opportunities before you retire, especially the catch-up contributions for investors age fifty-plus for tax-deferred employer plans and IRAs. Consolidate your retirement plans (e.g., IRAs) that are scattered among many financial providers.

GIVE YOURSELF A PAYCHECK

Let's say you did everything right and saved and invested as much as you could to prepare for your retirement, and you think your savings should be sufficient to carry you through. Still, you wouldn't be alone if you're worried about outliving your savings. But what if you could pay yourself every month with a retirement "paycheck" by withdrawing (no more than) 4 to 5 percent of your savings? If you are a conservative investor, you should consider withdrawing a lesser amount to be sure your money lasts as long as you do.

What You Need to Know

When you withdraw money for retirement income, start with taxable or tax-free investments, and allow tax-deferred accounts to grow as long as possible. Set aside a portion of your retirement savings for safer investments, such as CDs or money market mutual funds, to minimize your investment risk. The average expense on variable annuities is about 2 percent of assets. Shop around for low-cost providers with below-average expenses.

Here are several income sources to consider:

- **Pension Plans:** Benefits calculated based on earnings and years of employment
- **Plans:** Your employer's 401k, 403(b), and Section 457 plans are retirement accounts offered as an employee benefit
- **Individual Retirement Accounts (IRAs):** Tax-favored investment accounts that can be used to invest in stocks, bonds, mutual funds, electric funds transfers (EFTs), and other types of investments
- **Roth IRAs:** Contributions are made with after-tax dollars; any money generated within the Roth is never taxed again
- **SIMPLE IRAS** (Savings Incentive Match for Employees): A retirement plan that small businesses with up to one hundred employees can offer; works very much like a 401k
- **Taxable accounts:** Stocks, bonds, and mutual funds funded with after-tax savings
- **Proceeds from sales:** A home, rental real estate, and income from a reverse mortgage
- **Tax-free assets:** Municipal bonds (If possible, wait until age seventy-and-a-half to tap your tax-deferred accounts.)
- **Annuities:** Long-range investment with guaranteed lifetime income

- **Mutual funds:** Gradually shift portfolio investments into bonds or cash assets as you get older.

What You Need to Do

Ask yourself if you can really afford to retire. Do the math. If you've accumulated *ten times* your final pay in retirement savings, you probably can. Take advantage of tax-favored investments, such as Roth and/or traditional IRAs. Contribute as much as possible to your 401k or other tax-favored accounts at work. Consider consolidating all of your rollovers from 401k accounts into one or two accounts. If you roll them over into an IRA, you minimize the risk of your former employer going out of business or being acquired by another company.

WILLS AND ESTATE PLANNING

(This subject is covered in some detail in Chapter VII: "Talking to Your Adult Children" and Chapter X: "Facing End-of-Life Choices".) The thought of making a will may be unsettling, but it is important to do so while you are "of sound body and mind" to ensure that your money and property will go to those you want to have them after you're gone. Think of a will as a gift you give to loved ones. If you don't have a will, deciding who gets what can cause unnecessary hassles and delays, as well as the possibility of financial loss. Another reason to make a will now, while your mind is sharp, is that you—not the state probate court system—make decisions about what happens to your property.

What You Need to Know

Estate planning is necessary if you want your assets to be distributed according to your wishes with the lowest possible federal and state taxes. Your estate plan is not engraved in granite; it is fluid. As events occur in your life, such as being widowed or divorced or moving across the country, periodically review your planning documents and revise them to reflect the current reality. You should also regularly review the beneficiaries in your will, trusts, insurance policies, and retirement account.

If you die *intestate* (without a legal will), the state probate court will appoint an administrator to oversee and manage your estate. The administrator's duties include paying final expenses and distributing assets.

What You Need to Do

You need to play an active role in the estate-planning process, even if you have a professional helping you. Start by gathering and consolidating information about your personal property (e.g., bank statements, investment and retirement accounts, cars, jewelry, insurance policies, etc.). Let your children and your executor know where the original and copies are stored. Choose an executor to settle your estate according to your wishes. You might want two executors—a family member and an attorney with estate-planning expertise.

You should have these three estate-planning documents: a will, a living will for healthcare decisions, and a durable power of attorney for financial affairs. Hire a lawyer to prepare a will rather than write one on your own. To be valid, a will must comply strictly with state law. Update your will and power of attorney if and when circumstances change. Keeping a will current is just as important as drafting one in the first place. Regularly review the beneficiaries in your will, trusts, insurance policies, and retirement account. Another way to make sure your assets are professionally managed is to establish a trust, particularly for minors or older children who are unable to care for themselves.

Bill Hosner

An Active Investor

Bill Hosner had a couple of advantages growing up: his parents. His father was an accountant and his mother a mathematician. All his life he learned the value of numbers, and numbers equated to money. He and his siblings were taught how to save money, which was a gift in itself. He made his first investment at the age of sixteen and became instantly hooked on investing. After earning a business degree in management and marketing from Southeast Missouri State, his first job was as a manufacturer's rep for an HVAC company. Eventually, he became the owner of the company. He sold the company in 2018 and became a full-time investor.

◆　◆　◆

It's wise to begin investing your money as soon as you can, and the best place to earn a good return on your money is in the stock market. When your money starts making money for you, you can have a nice monthly income.

In the 2008 recession, people claimed they lost money. However, that only happened if they pulled their money out of the market. It's true that those who left their money in the market could have seen anywhere between a 30 to 40 percent drop; but in 2010-2011, they would have seen about a 45 percent gain, which would have nullified their previous loss. We have seen the market fluctuate daily, monthly, and yearly, as it did in the early1990s and the early 2000s. The DOW and the market will always reflect the current state of the economy. The DOW averages 10 percent a year over time. Some years it will be lower, and some years it will be higher. So, it's best not to panic and pull your investments out if the stock market crashes.

If the market does have a downward turn, however, realigning some of your investments to include the companies for which there is a strong need in the economy and that will rebound is a smart move. In other words, moving your money around in the market to invest in stocks that are more than likely to go up is a good idea.

If you have your money in big companies, such as Disney or Boeing or Marriott, the only way you're going to lose money is if the company goes bankrupt, and those companies are not going to go bankrupt. Their stocks may go down during downtimes, but they're going to come right back up to where they were and potentially climb even higher. It happens all the time.

You can also earn income if you have whole-life insurance, which is an investment that has a cash value you can borrow from at a reasonable interest rate. You're putting in money on a regular basis, and the insurance company is also investing that money. So, your money is growing along with the insurance company's investments, although not at a very rapid rate, for several years. The insurance company is investing your money in order to earn enough over time to pay the face value of your insurance policy upon your death.

If you have term-life insurance, let's say you're going to pay $1,000 a year. As long as you pay, your policy is in force; when you stop paying, it's gone. There is nothing left. There are some companies that will buy your term-life insurance policy, but this is only beneficial for an older policy holder. The company will continue making the payments, but when you pass away, the company becomes the beneficiary.

Reverse mortgages are another way to earn income. There are myriad types of reverse mortgages. Your options could be to borrow against your house, take a lump sum payment, or be paid monthly. If you own a house and you have equity in the house, and if you feel you have fewer than ten years of life left, a reverse mortgage might be a good solution. If you think you have twenty years left, a reverse mortgage probably isn't beneficial. Upon your death, the lender will own your house and will have the freedom to rent or sell it. You do not have to pay back the money the lender has paid you. There will be an exclusion in the contract specifying how many years you will continue to be paid. If you are in your eighties and in good health, this probably wouldn't be a good option for you now.

A lot of older people put their money in Certificates of Deposit (CDs), which will pay you 1 to 1.5 percent. That's it. $100,000 is going to make you $1,500 a year. The bank is investing your money in the market. If you invest that money in the market yourself, the market may have a down year or two, but it's always going to come back. Putting your money in the market, in my opinion, is always the safe way to go.

If the question is what should you *not* invest in, the answer is CDs. If you like the idea of a guaranteed amount, you can buy bonds, which will pay you 5 percent, maybe as high as 7 percent. A bond assures you of a 98 percent payback. The only way the company can get out of paying you is if it goes bankrupt. This is not the best option if you need money quickly because you cannot keep pulling your money out of a bond. Most bonds pay out for five or ten years. You can't touch your initial principle for a couple of years, but you can receive the interest on the bond either monthly or quarterly.

I've talked to a lot of younger people about investments, and they often tell me they don't have any money. Yet, they will have a $200 cable bill, or they are driving around in a Lexus or some other expensive car. They wouldn't think about getting rid of cable, but that's money they could put towards an investment or paying off something they owe. They could get a less-expensive car, but that's not something many people are willing to do. If you have a house, there are real estate taxes, which can be very high. If you have a car, there is a car payment, upkeep, insurance, and taxes. Even if you cut expenses when you're older, you can slash hundreds off your monthly bills.

In a nutshell, my advice is this:

1. Buy whole-life insurance, which allows you to borrow from or sell your insurance for a cash value.
2. If you have money, invest in the stock market and/or buy bonds. I recommend that you don't put your money into CDs.
3. If possible, live with a family member until you get your financial situation worked out.
4. Drive a less-expensive car, get rid of cable, pay off credit cards, and think of all the ways you could cut expenses.

5. A reverse mortgage is your last option, and you shouldn't do that unless you think you're close to the end of your life.

Paul Lang*
An ER Physician's Assistant

Paul Lang is a physician's assistant (PA) in the field of cardiology. He graduated from the University of Florida in 1982 with a bachelor's degree in medicine. His first job was as a Navy corpsman. He has been in the field of medicine for thirty-eight years. At sixty-six, he is thinking about retirement and plans to stop working in four years, at seventy. By that time, his wife, who is eight years younger than he, will be eligible for social security. From a financial standpoint, that should work out well. To live where they want to live, he and his wife are building a new house closer to the beach than they are now.
*Name has been changed to protect the interviewee's identity.

When you're thinking about retiring, the first question you have to ask yourself is, *Who are you?* If you say, *Well, I'm a doctor,* that's what you *do,* not who you *are.* You're no longer going to be doing what you do. Are you Carl, the fisherman ... Carl, the artist ... Carl, the walker ... Carl, the gym rat? If you define yourself by your profession, and you are no longer in your profession when you retire, then you don't have an identity.

What I learned from being off for three weeks because of COVID-19 is that I'm not ready to retire. And when I am ready, I'm going to have to transition into retirement and not just stop working. Maybe I will work less but not completely stop working.

Here are three more questions I think are worth considering before you accept the proverbial gold watch: *Do you have enough? Have you had enough? Do you have enough to do?* If you answered yes to all three, you're probably ready to retire.

I ran into a guy who was a pharmaceutical rep. He said, in planning his retirement, both from a financial standpoint and from a what-are-you-going-to-do standpoint, he looked at what to expect in the coming years. As you get older, first, you have your go-go years when you're still young enough, strong enough, and healthy enough to go. You travel, take vacations, visit family, go fishing or hunting or skiing or whatever you want to do.

Then you have your slow-go years, when you still go, but your activities are less demanding than those you engaged in during your go-go years. Instead of hiking, you may opt for taking a walk in the park or going to museums. You can still go, but you are slowing down.

Finally you have your no-go years, when your mobility decreases and you may have physical or mental impairments, so you don't go. You're going to have to start planning for those years. Where are you going to live? What are you going to be able to do? How much support are you going to need?

That was one way of looking at retirement. My brother, Matt, is going to be sixty-two in July of 2022. The day he turns sixty-two he's going to retire. The day after that he is going to hook up his Airstream and drive to the Grand Canyon. He already has his plan. My brother, Mark, retired and decided he wanted to go back to work. Now he's working part time. My older brother, John, is retired and can't believe he got everything done that he's doing now when he was working.

I think the biggest mistake people make when it comes to money for retirement is not starting to save when they are young. For many people who are living paycheck to paycheck, there's no money left to save. People who are fortunate enough to save may be saving for their kids' education, or for an emergency, or for a house. But they aren't saving for retirement. It doesn't even occur to them, because when you're twenty-five, it's hard to imagine yourself at sixty-five. I worked two jobs to save enough money for my kids' college funds. I did not have a 401k from my employer at that time, but I got one later and took full advantage of it.

Ideally, you should save 10 percent of your salary for retirement and more if you can. If you're young enough, you can save 10 percent one year, 11 percent the following year, 12 percent the year after that, and so on. Assuming that your earnings are growing as well, by the end of ten years, you're saving 20 percent, which is ideal. The more you save and invest, the more your money will grow.

The other thing I learned from my parents and their retirement is that you have to adjust your lifestyle. They are very happy with their lifestyle. They don't travel; they don't take vacations, though occasionally they will take a cruise or visit family. They are eighty-five and eighty-seven, and they are in their no-go years. They're still independent, but in terms of getting through an airport or taking a long car ride —no. Up until about three years ago, they had a summer place in North Carolina, and they would go there from May through September and then spend the other part of the year here in Florida.

The last time they did that, they were driving back from North Carolina to Florida, and they nearly got into an accident on the interstate. They were so shaken up that they had to pull over to the side of the road. They made the decision then and there that neither one of them felt comfortable driving long distances on the highway anymore. They realized that they had limitations. That's not to say that they gave up driving. They still take short day trips, but they don't take any long driving trips anymore or drive at night. They've adjusted their lifestyle.

They have a close group of friends they play cards with. They don't like going to movies. They prefer to eat at home, so they don't go out to restaurants a lot. After they are out shopping, they may go to a little Italian restaurant they like a lot for lunch. They go out for coffee with friends, and my dad plays cards with a few guys three times a week.

I've heard that you need 80 percent of your gross income to live in retirement with your current lifestyle. The ideal is to retire debt-free, so you don't have a mortgage or outstanding debt. Our financial advisors told us that for his higher-income-earning clients, 80 percent is not necessary. I read somewhere that if you make $75,000 a year, that's enough for food, clothing, and some entertainment. For some people, that's going to require a lifestyle adjustment. I couldn't fathom some of the physicians I know living on $75,000 a year. If you're making $500,000 a year, do you really need $400,000 a year to live? No, I don't think so. So, the 80 percent doesn't always apply.

I think your attitude about retirement starts with the numbers—the money. Then, to make the numbers work, it's not an attitude about money; it's an attitude about life. It should be whatever is right for you. I want to have enough money so that I don't have to worry about food, clothing, and shelter. And I want to have enough money to travel. I don't have to travel the globe, but every year or every other year, I would like to take a big vacation—perhaps two weeks to Europe. If my children are living away, I want to be able to go visit them. But to rent an RV and spend two months driving across the country is not for me.

I have always had a desire or a dream to live by the water—not the ocean, but a lake—and wake up in the morning and walk out onto the deck and see the sunrise. In talking to people who do live near water, they say it looks like a glamorous life but that there's a lot of work, especially in Florida with storms and flooding and damage to their docks. I knew a psychiatrist who lived close to the water and liked to fish. His license plate said Fish Doctor. Every year he went to Michigan or someplace up North to fish. I told him I had always wanted to live near water. And he said, you should live where you want to live just because you want to live there, not because you think oh, it would be a good financial investment to live in a high-rise high rise in Manhattan.

We're building a new house. We want to live in a community that, during our go-go years and our slow-go years, we can step out the door and walk to the grocery store, walk to a restaurant, walk to the library, or take public transportation. There is a website where you can look up a neighborhood or community and see its walkability score for whether you can walk somewhere or get in your car to go there. If we want to go to a restaurant or for a walk or to ride our bikes, we don't want to have to get in our car to go to where we want to be. Where we live now is a very nice neighborhood, but if you even want to go to a local coffee shop, you have to get in your car and go.

When my daughter lived in Boston and in Cambridge, she loved living where she lived. She could walk to the dry cleaner, she could walk to her favorite coffee shop, and she could walk around the corner to the grocery store. Here, if you're cooking dinner and you suddenly realize you need a spice or some other ingredient, you have to get in your car and drive three miles to the grocery store and then drive three miles home. That's where the new house fits in.

My wife wants to build a house where people will come to visit. Not to be negative or morbid, but you really don't know what the next day is going to bring, particularly now. I heard someone on NPR talking about the current pandemic situation. He said he and his wife own a cabin somewhere up North. They are older, and he's had asthma most of his life. He said, "If I get COVID, it's likely to be a death sentence for me." So he and his wife decided early on that they would go and live in their cabin. The only person he's been in contact with, other than on Zoom, has been his wife. He said he wondered about people like him who are older and with health problems in quarantine. Are their final days going to be in quarantine? Is that how their lives will end? "We never expected anything like this," he said. "We were socially active people. We had friends over; we had parties. And now we are quarantined. I ask myself, is this the way *my* life will end?"

You don't know what's going to happen. I see patients who are fine one day and not the next. Some are relatively young; some are older. Yes, you should live in the moment, but you have to plan for the future. You hope you will have a long and healthy life. Everyone's goal is to live as long as they can and as well as they can. What they want to shorten is that time in their lives where they're living, but they're not well. They want what we all want—quality of life.

IX. BUILDING YOUR SUPPORT SYSTEM

How will you build and maintain your social circle?

IF YOU HAVE FOUND that the older you get, the harder it is to make new friends, believe me—you are not alone. All the ways in which we made friends when we were younger don't apply to our current stage of life. We aren't attending consciousness-raising groups, going to Jazzercise, or pushing baby carriages down the street (that's how we got around back then). Some of our old friends have either drifted away or become ill; perhaps *we* have drifted away as well without realizing it. Staying in touch with people who are no longer part of our lives takes a lot of energy and motivation.

As more and more people work from home, it is easy to become isolated. I certainly did. Writing is a solitary vocation, and doing it in a home office for thirty years is not conducive to meeting people. I never realized how much time I was spending alone until I retired.

We need friends all our lives but never more than in our later years. According to Abraham Maslow, "Humans need to love and be loved ... Many people become susceptible to loneliness, social anxiety, and clinical depression in the absence of this love or belonging." Research from Brigham Young University concludes that having a dwindling social circle or not having enough close friends has a similar risk factor as smoking fifteen cigarettes per day.

"Friends become increasingly important to health and happiness as people age," says an article in *Personal Relationships*. "They're so crucial, in fact, that having supportive friendships in old age was found to be a stronger predictor of well-being than having strong family connections." Relationships account for more than 70 percent of our happiness.

A *Journal of Health and Social Behavior* report published in 2010 noted that having strong social bonds helps us live longer. It boosts our immune system and allows us to enjoy a more meaningful life. Strong friendships can help to reduce stress, chronic pain, the risk of heart disease, and high blood pressure. These are all good reasons to make friends.

The importance of friendships in later life is of great interest to professionals who deal with the elderly. For example, William Chopik, assistant professor of psychology at Michigan State University, analyzed a survey of nearly 7,500 older people in the United States. He found that it wasn't only important to have friends but that the quality of those friendships mattered just as much.

But Chopik says the power of friendship on physical and mental health is often ignored in research—especially in older people, where relationships with spouses and children are considered more important. And yet some studies show that we often enjoy our time with friends more than we do with family. Of course, some people are lucky enough to share powerful friendships with members of their immediate family. I can certainly attest to that, since my best friends are my sister and my daughters. "The important thing is having people you can rely on, for the good times as well as the bad," notes Chopik.

We not only need friends, but we need those friends to be part of our support system. Life is unpredictable, especially as we grow older. When we hit a rough patch, we need those who will understand what we are going through or at least be able to listen to us as we try to explain. A support system is more than just a group of people to bounce ideas off of. These people become what is referred to in business as a "mastermind group" who will share their own thoughts and give us feedback on ours (Gail Gardner in *Small Trends Business*, Feb. 2020).

Although they had no name for their conversations, people have participated in mastermind groups for as long as they have communicated with each other. But it wasn't until 1925, when Napoleon Hill gave these gatherings a name, that the term caught on. In his best-selling book, *Think and Grow Rich*, Hill defined a mastermind group as "a peer-to-peer mentoring gathering used to help members solve their problems with input and advice from the other group members." That sounds a lot like the support system described above.

This never occurred to us when we were younger, unless we were in a business setting—so why is this something we need in our seventies, eighties, and nineties? We need it because giving and receiving support from others is a basic human need. We need it because having a support system leads to higher levels of well-being, better coping skills, and a longer and healthier life. As an added bonus, we needed because it also reduces depression and anxiety.

How to Begin

If you want to develop a support network, start by looking around you. Who is in your life? Some of them are already your friends—people who care about you, are willing to listen to you, and give you sage advice when you ask for it. If you are honest with yourself, there are also people in your life who bring you down. Perhaps they are going through a rough time in their own lives, or they may be consistently negative for reasons you can't possibly know. These are not the kind of people you would invite to be part of your support system because they can drain your energy, which is the opposite of what you want.

So where do you find the people who will energize you and be there for you when you need them? First, think a little bit about the kind of people with whom you want to surround yourself. Then take inventory of your friends and decide who fits in your ideal group. Don't limit yourself to only people you know because this is a perfect opportunity for you to meet new people by pursuing your passions and finding others who are already doing what you love. You might join a book club or take a class at your gym or get active in your place of worship or political party. This way, you will be meeting people who already share some of your interests.

Have an open mind. Expose yourself to new situations, new opportunities, and new people you will meet along the way. If you recall, when you were much younger, you and your friends tended to think alike, dress alike, and even look alike. Sometimes it may have felt as if you were all stamped out of the same cookie-cutter. What was once a pretty homogeneous world is far more interesting now. You are likely to meet people who don't think like you or dress like you, and they certainly don't look like you.

Being open to new opportunities often means stepping outside your comfort zone. When a new friend invites you go somewhere you have never been or do something you have never done, and you're tempted to say no thank you, pause a few seconds to reconsider. You might actually have fun, but if you refuse too often, the invitations may stop coming.

Another way to meet new people who share your values is to volunteer for a cause you care about, such as a charity, civic organization, or a political campaign you want to support. You won't love everyone you meet, of course, but you might make a friend or two. At the very least, you will be contributing your time to a cause that is important to you.

If you join your local gym, you probably won't meet people by limiting yourself to solitary pursuits, such as the treadmill or resistance machines. You need to take a class or two. There are so many benefits to working out with others: learning new exercises, meeting new people, and having someone to compete with besides yourself. For those who are computer savvy, check out friendship apps that will allow you to meet new people from across the street, across the country, and across the world. Apps like Meetup, MeetMe, Revel-Social, Nextdoor, and Bumble are worth exploring.

Connecting with strangers online can feel a bit intimidating, but if you approach it with the right attitude, the effort can lead you to some great friendships that might last a lifetime. You can also search for like-minded people online by checking out hashtags you find interesting or related to things you enjoy doing or want to know more about.

While a circle of friends is ideal, there are many other sources of support: family, neighbors, clergy, therapists, and even pets. Pets are the perfect antidote to loneliness. Dogs, particularly, are there for you 24/7. They love you unconditionally. Smaller dogs can easily travel with you wherever you go, not to mention their cuddle factor.

Finally, here are some quick tips from Theo Harrison at *Your Tang* on how to make friends:

- Visit unfamiliar sites in your city.
- Connect with the coworkers you like.
- Reach out to your neighbors.
- Join a meetup group, and participate actively.
- Join a book club, or start one.
- Start or join an online group.
- Take part in a sports league.
- Get a dog and walk around your neighborhood.
- Research and attend networking events.
- Take a class in a subject that interests you.

Once you have made some new friends, it's up to you to keep those friendships alive and thriving. That means taking the initiative to stay in touch and get together. Over the years, I have discovered that some of the friends I treasure most are least likely to pick up the phone and suggest coffee or dinner. I am usually the one to call. It used to bother me, but who calls whom no longer seems important—only that we see each other now and then.

When you talk to a close friend, it's tempting to tell the person your problems, but that's not what friendship is supposed to be about. If you find yourself doing that too often, try asking your friend what's happening in her life or what's on her mind. Tune in to her facial expressions and body language; you'll know if there is something she wants to talk about. Women are particularly good about reading these cues; men have to work a little harder at it but are usually quick studies.

Everything worth doing takes effort. And nothing is worthier of that effort than making friends and building a support network in which people are there for you when you need them, and you are there for them. Support is a two-way street. True friends will go the extra mile for you and expect nothing in return. But to be a true friend, you must be willing to reciprocate. If you have gotten in the habit of doing so earlier in your life, this will come naturally to you. Friendship is a gift you give yourself as well as those you befriend.

Why You Need an Advocate

In addition to a group of friends you can depend on, you are doubly blessed if you also have family members who love you and will do everything possible to keep you healthy and safe. As your needs increase over time, the things your adult children do for you increase as well. Often, the more they help, the more tightly you cling to your autonomy. I certainly tried to remain as independent as possible, for as long as possible, even when it was clear that some activities were becoming harder for me to handle. I wanted to do the things I had always done and fill every role I had mastered in the past.

There was one role, however, that I was unable to assume: that of advocate. An advocate is someone who speaks on your behalf in situations where you may be uncomfortable doing so, are unable to do so, or don't have the requisite knowledge of the subject. In short, an advocate goes to bat for you when you can't do it yourself. If you've ever been in the hospital for any reason, you probably realized that it was important to have someone who made sure you were getting the care and attention you needed. My daughters were my advocates on more than one occasion.

There are two types of advocates: one who focuses on your health and one who oversees your finances. One or more of your children can take on these responsibilities if they are willing to do so, if they live in the same city as you do, and if they are comfortable dealing with medical and financial professionals.

There are many reasons why your children or other family members may not be the best choices to fill this role. If that is the case, you can hire someone to advocate on your behalf. The best way to find the right person is to ask people you already know at your bank or some other financial institution for a recommendation. Your primary care doctor or any specialist you see is also an excellent source of referrals, as are any of your friends who have an advocate they like and trust.

Health advocates do not have to be medical professionals, but they must be able to communicate equally well with you and your doctors. Your health advocate can help you navigate the medical system by:

- Identifying physicians, specialists, and hospitals that meet your needs as an older adult and are covered by your insurance plan
- Helping you complete your medical history forms for doctors and hospital stays
- Scheduling appointments and accompanying you to doctors' appointments, asking pertinent questions, and ensuring that all of your concerns are addressed
- Keeping track of your symptoms, the effectiveness of current treatments, and any issues doctors should be aware of
- Dealing with health insurance companies on such subjects as what is covered, claims billing, and payments
- Giving your doctors an overview of your medical situation, coordinating treatments, and helping to find solutions to any side effects that may occur

- Managing your current medications, ensuring that drugs and supplements are reviewed regularly, and being aware of any potential drug interactions
- Explaining clearly what you should know about your health conditions, treatments, prescriptions, and your doctor's instructions
- Keeping in touch with nursing staff in assisted-living facilities to facilitate communication among your doctors, your family, the facility, and you

Managing your money can sometimes feel like getting lost in a maze. Financial advocates can clear the path by:

- Acting on your behalf as a trustee, personal representative, or power of attorney
- Helping you balance your checkbook, keep track of your bank account, and pay bills on time or through automatic deduction
- Acting as agents to secure Social Security benefits
- Preparing tax returns for you, your estate, and your trust
- Setting up required minimum distributions from IRA accounts
- Providing financial advisor oversight to be sure your assets are being managed as you had intended
- Offering financial advice and assistance regarding medical and other types of bills
- Acting as a liaison between you and your insurance companies
- Handling financial obligations so that you and your physicians can focus on healthcare

---

Benita Crook
An Advocate for the Elderly

Benita was a co-owner of a private-duty nursing company for almost twenty years. After seeing that some patient needs could not be met by the agency, she started Senior Care Advocates eight years ago. Her primary clients are those without a family or with a family unable or unwilling to help. To meet the needs of clients, she works closely with trust officers, case managers, and elder-care lawyers in the St. Louis area. Benita serves on the board of HOPE, an organization dedicated to affordable housing needs for seniors. She has lived in St. Louis since 1978 and has two adult children, four grandchildren, and two adorable rescue cats.

I ran a private-duty nursing agency for many years, and what prompted me to start my business was that I discovered there were a lot of things we could not do. We could not get sufficient information from the doctor for clients because clients didn't think aides were capable of getting the right information. We couldn't help people pay their bills because of the conflict of interest. It was pretty obvious that people needed help with these things. Care managers, at that time, were just starting up and were the only people the family could contact. We could not help with power of attorney or much of what care managers could do.

When I left the private-duty business, I realized that advocacy was a needed service. I get a lot of referrals from care managers because the work I do frees them up to handle other things. A case manager is usually a social worker but sometimes a nurse. They know the ins and outs of the system and about programs, how to qualify for money from the government, and good and bad nursing homes.

I took a marketing approach to the business: What is the need, and how can I meet that need with my experience, tools, knowledge, connections, etc.? So that's exactly what I did. I started calling my contacts—people who had known me from my private-duty business and even before that. A trust officer or an eldercare lawyer called me and asked if I would consider being a power of attorney or a trustee for estates where people didn't have anyone.

An example of a good use of an advocate is my client who has three children, all of whom live out of town. I am the go-between for them. I take the client to the doctor, send her children an email about the visit, and take care of any discrepancies when her bills come in.

When I have the power of attorney and am in charge of somebody's estate, I first meet with the people to make sure they agree to work with me. I find out about their circumstances so I can be aware of problems down the line with their family members. Then, I provide them with a list of questions: Who has access to your safe deposit box? Where are the keys? Do you have pets that need to be taken care of? Do you have a trust? Is everything in the trust's name? These are things they may not have thought about—because who thinks about those things?

I tell clients to get their ducks in a row while they're conscious and coherent, because if they don't do all these things now, they are not going to have another chance to do it later. You can't put a power of attorney in place if you're deemed mentally unstable. I now have power of attorney for fifteen people. So if I have your power of attorney, and you have to go to the hospital, I meet you there because I have all your information.

Power of attorney for healthcare only deals with healthcare issues. I can make doctors' appointments, talk to doctors, and make sure prescriptions are filled. Most of the time clients indicate whether they want to be resuscitated or not. If you want to be sure you will not be resuscitated, you should have something called an out of hospital DNR form. (A DNR wrist band is purple; a DNR printed document is yellow.) If there is a DNR, EMTs need to know that before they get there. The form contains the name of a contact person, your power of attorney, and your doctor. If it's someplace visible, where paramedics can find it, they can call and clarify the DNR.

If I'm going to act as a power of attorney, there is an upfront fee, and then you pay nothing else until I have to take action. An advocate will make sure you are represented at doctors' appointments, with your family, and at facilities. She sees to it that your bills are paid and works with case managers. I can go with you to the doctor, talk to the doctor about what the issues are, make sure you have an up-to-date medication list at those appointments, and help doctors determine if any adjustments need to be made. Then, if family members are involved, I send them an email that explains what we did in the doctor's office. If a family member has the power of attorney and some crisis occurs, I don't make the decision; the family member does. If that person can't get here, she can call the doctor or hospital and grant permission for me to do whatever is required.

A power of attorney for financial matters can pay bills and sell your house if you are incapacitated. I can do just about anything you would do. Clients find me through their bank; the trust officer who handles their money; their eldercare lawyer if they have a good one; a friend who has used me in the past; or, if they live in assisted living or a nursing home, the facility management will call me.

The generation of people who are in their eighties and nineties typically pay their bills as soon as they arrive. They don't look to see whether the bill has already been paid or if it has been submitted to the insurance company. They just pay it. When I'm working with my clients, I go over all of that. If I see that the bill has not been submitted to Medicare, I call and ask why it has not been submitted. If they don't have somebody doing that, older people will just pay those bills. If they go into the hospital, the biggest thing the advocate can do is be there, talk to the staff, and make regular visits. It's important for hospital staff to know that someone is going to be there. The same is true in nursing homes. An advocate in facilities can be a positive go-between for clients and staff. Families get relief knowing someone is there when they can't be.

I learned a lot about what I do by working with case managers over the years and from being a long-term care ombudsman. Most of what

I do is common sense: How would I want to be treated? How would I want my mother to be treated? That's how I usually make my decisions.

If you don't have an advocate, you may personally have to work with hospital case managers. People who don't have an advocate or someone to help them can flounder. You may end up in a nursing home you don't like or one that doesn't meet your needs.

Being a trustee comes into play when a person passes and the estate needs to be disbursed. A recent client passed away, and she had no relatives in town. As a trustee, it was my job to separate her household items, give some to charity, sell her car and her home, clean out her safe deposit box, sell her jewelry, and contact a lawyer and all of her beneficiaries.

Advice to Older People

Stay active as long as you can, make your own decisions as long as you can, and try to recognize when you are beginning to feel you can't make good decisions. That's when you need an advocate. You may not want your adult children to have control over your life. You may not want to tell them everything, but somebody should have that information. That somebody is your advocate.

Criteria for a Good Advocate

Here are the important questions to ask:

- Is this person able to listen to your issues with an open mind and not start giving you answers before she hears the whole story?
- Is she willing to talk openly with you, and if there are children involved, to listen to their perspective? The advocate can look at the big picture and see all sides of the story, as sometimes things become very clear when you have the whole picture.
- Is this person flexible because you don't know when you're going to the hospital or when you might need somebody to help you for longer than the scheduled time?

- Is this a person who doesn't say no to a client?
- Does she take a holistic approach to you and your issues?
- Is this person organized, especially when it comes to handling client estates?
- Can she empathize with you? She can't approach this job like a business; she has to be like a family member.

Janell Nunn
Creating Her Own Support Network

Janell Nunn is the mother of two daughters, the grandmother of four grandchildren, a tennis player, an all-around athlete, and someone who can't stand to be stuck indoors. After her divorce, she realized her social circle was made up of her husband's friends and coworkers—so she set out to create a new one. Tennis became not only her avocation but the source of close friends and an enduring support system. Though she insists she doesn't "hold onto people," her early, post-divorce friendships have lasted for years.

Before my divorce, which was something I didn't want, our friends were kind of his friends. We belonged to a country club. He was a golfer; I wasn't a golfer. He also had his work friends. I told myself I didn't need friends. I had him. But I remember thinking, *You know, I really don't have anyone where I could say I am coming over with a glass of wine*, but I didn't do that anyway. I had kids. I was the perfect mother. Yet I think I felt like something was missing because a lot of people in St. Louis got together with their friends who had known each other since grammar school. I didn't have that because I didn't grow up here.

I'm not introverted; I just don't invest myself in people. I don't let them know me or what I'm feeling. I would never let people know anything I thought would disappoint them. I guess I'm not a deep-feeling person.

After the divorce, I knew I wasn't going to keep any of our friends as my friends. I could call the women to do things with, and they did include me the first year or two in some aspects of their social life. I think some of them liked me more than they liked my husband. As it turns out, that was true, but I didn't know that then.

I was a dental hygienist and worked three days a week. I saw my chance to make friends would be through tennis, which I did play. I started playing more with USTA (United States Tennis Association). To this day, 80 percent of my friends are from tennis. Many of them are easily ten years younger than I am. Some of the people I played with years ago don't play anymore, as they have injuries or have aged out. I'm aging out right now at seventy-one. I don't play as well as I did twenty years ago, but I'm still a good player and still enjoy it.

I made it a cause to make friends after my divorce. Another tennis player was also getting divorced, and she introduced me to another tennis player who was doing it, too. We were going to divorce-recovery groups, and even though we were in separate groups at separate times, we would get our groups together for outings. Then I had another friend whose kids had gone to school with my kids since kindergarten, and she was also going through a divorce. We were all hurting, and we would get together and talk—a lot. That's the first time I ever had true friends, and we are still friends to this day. I would say they were my saving grace. We traveled; we went to other countries. One friend had a boat that we kept using even though it was her soon-to-be-ex-husband's boat.

I won't talk to just anyone, but sometimes I think, *That looks like a fun group. I'm going to try to meet them and maybe become friends.* You have to make an effort, and I do. I have a group that goes to plays. We go to the Rep, the Fox, and the Stray Dog Theater. We have that common interest, and we are all tennis players. I'll look to see what's going on in St. Louis, and often I'll think, *I'd like to do that,* or *I want to try that restaurant.* Who would I call to go with me? Sometimes I do think maybe I should have a man in my life, so we could go to that expensive restaurant or a brewery hop or something like that. It would be easier sometimes to have a husband to do things with.

I've had a rather well-rounded life, and my bucket list is pretty empty right now. I only regret that the family didn't stay together, but I don't regret not being with my ex-husband. I've been divorced twenty-one years. I did date, and one stuck for a while. I was pretty picky, and I wasn't desperate for a man. I have friends who are, and they're probably going to find one. When I meet some of the people they have found, I think, *Oh, I couldn't spend five minutes with that person.*

I am really active, and not doing things now (during this pandemic) is driving me crazy. I walk sometimes twice a day. I don't sit still well. The other day it rained, and I was ready to go outside and scream. I do communicate with my friends on the phone and Zoom, but not as much as we did before. Now it's all texting.

I think that in order to make a life that's fulfilling, friends are very important. I just saw something on *CBS This Morning* about loneliness in the elderly. It's a huge thing, and this doctor said that being consistently lonely—experiencing that deep, deep loneliness when you don't have friends and you don't know how to find them—is like smoking fifteen cigarettes a day in terms of your health.

I am an organizer, so, I'll say, *Who wants to go to such and such?* And all of a sudden, I'll have seven people going. If you wait to let someone else take the initiative, you may wait a long time. I have one friend who I swore to myself I was going to wait until she called me to do something, and I'm still waiting. I've even said to her, "If there is something you want to do, all you have to do is call me, and I'll probably be interested." Yet in twenty-some years, she has never called me with the plan. She does call, but she wants to know what I'm doing so she can hop in. She's someone who is desperate for a man.

I was popular in high school, but I didn't have those deep friendships some people had. I know people who have stayed in touch with friends from high school. I can't imagine doing that. What would I have in common with someone I haven't seen since I was eighteen? I think it would be difficult at this age to go out and start making new friends again. My friendships now are based on shared interests, which works for me.

X. FACING END-OF-LIFE CHOICES

How do you make your wishes known and fulfilled?

Like every other species on earth, we have a finite amount of time on this planet. Our lives will end; that's a given. We stare death in the face every day in the news, in violent movies and TV shows, and in some places, up close and personal. We know this is how our stories will end, and yet, in our culture, we seem to be in a state of perpetual denial. Death happens all around us, but on some level, we cling to the hope that it will not happen to us. Death will come, of course, so the only logical approach for us is to be better prepared for the inevitable last chapter in our lives. Preparation means facing reality and taking the necessary steps to let those who are close to us know what we hope for in our final days.

Because we are a society fixated on death from a distance, many people wait until they are terminally ill or in a life-threatening situation before they confront end-of-life decisions and plans. Of course, facing them is never easy, but we should do so while we are still thinking clearly and able to articulate our desires. No matter how ready we may be to identify our needs ahead of time, we are bound to feel a whole range of emotions, including shock, fear, or guilt about being a burden to loved ones. Nearing the end of your life may be a difficult time for you and for your family. Whatever feelings you are having, just know that they are normal. Some of the powerful emotions you can expect to have include:

Fear

Although it's not unusual to be afraid to die, understanding exactly what part of dying you fear might help. Are you afraid you will be alone or in pain; that your life had no purpose or meaning; or that the idea of heaven is a myth, and there is nothing beyond earthly life? If you know what you are afraid of, you will have an easier time managing your fear and helping others understand what you are dealing with. If you share your feelings with your family and medical team, they can find ways to ease some of your fears.

Anger

Very few people feel ready to die. It's perfectly normal to feel angry about your life ending—maybe earlier than you expected. You may lash out, often at those closest to you, but try instead to direct your anger at the disease or condition and not at your loved ones. You could also channel your anger as a source of energy to help you take action where it is called for.

Guilt and Regret

In the last stage of life, you might feel guilty about things you have done or not done, or something you have said. You might feel regret when you think that you should have done something differently or not done at all. But neither guilt nor regret will undo what's been done or said. Sometimes, the best course is to forgive yourself for things that are out of your control. This is a good time to talk with your children about how to handle *their* feelings and the loss they will soon go through.

Grief

To feel intense grief during the last stage of your life is a natural reaction.

You're grieving the loss of the life you planned and expected. You may already have lost the strength to get around as well as you used to, or the interest in doing the things you once enjoyed, or maybe the ability to get together with friends. Remember that the people you love are grieving, too. They know they're about to physically lose you. The good that can come from facing your grief together is realizing how much you mean to each other. It's never too late to do that.

Anxiety and Depression

Anxiety shows up in various forms: a nervous stomach, a shaky feeling all over, dread or worry, or fear of the unknown. Some anxiety is expected, but if you are experiencing severe symptoms, you might want to consider counseling or medication. The goal is to make you more comfortable and help you better cope with the changes taking place at this time in your life.

Depression is more than just feeling sad. The sadness could last for weeks or even months. You may feel hopeless or helpless, useless, and melancholy. You will no longer take joy in activities you once loved. These feelings make this time even harder than it has to be. Managing anxiety and depression well can make a big difference in your quality of life.

Feeling Alone

When you know you are nearing the end, you may feel a profound sense of loneliness that happens even when people are around you. Often, people on your care team can talk to you in a way that helps you feel less lonely. Some of them, such as hospice social workers, nurses, or other caregivers, may be experts in helping people at the end of their lives. They have that special gift for silence and the ability to listen when that is what you need. Finding people with whom you can connect can ease your sense of loneliness. Your healthcare team may be one of your greatest resources in this area.

Seeking Meaning

As human beings, we need meaning in our lives. We are hardwired to seek a reason for being here and for what has happened to us along the way. Viktor Frankl's *Man's Search for Meaning* has been called one of the ten most influential books in America. In it, Frankl argues that we cannot avoid suffering, but we can choose how to cope with it, find meaning in it, and move forward with renewed purpose. People find meaning in many different ways—some, in their work; others, in raising a family; still others, in their creative endeavors. Maybe you're wondering what your special contribution to the world has been; or perhaps you would like your children, family, and friends to remember you in a certain way. The end-of-life experience is full of meaning that can be uncovered through personal reflection. Sharing your thoughts, experiences, and wisdom is a gift your friends and family can cherish for years to come.

Making Your Wishes Known

I've already described the documents you need to have on hand and in a safe place that your family members know about. As I mentioned in Chapter VII: "Talking to Your Adult Children," the essential documents are a will, advanced directives or a living will, a durable power of attorney for healthcare, and your preferences about your funeral and/or memorial service. Filling out those documents takes a lot of introspection and self-reflection. If you are completing them with a partner or spouse, sit down and talk through every important point so that you both understand what the other person wants—and be willing to firmly advocate for them if necessary.

These four essential documents, which you might want to have drawn up by an attorney, are legally binding. They are witnessed and notarized and an accurate depiction of your desires. There are many things to think about at a time when you might be least able to do so, which is why it's so important to take the time now to talk through what you will want later.

Other Personal Wishes

Besides the provisions of these legal documents, you may have other wishes about end-of-life care, such as how you want people to treat you, how you wish to be made comfortable, and what you want your loved ones to know. There is an instrument that allows you to express all of these desires, as well as those in the above documents, and is legally binding in the District of Columbia and forty-two states. *Five Wishes* is a living will that addresses your personal, emotional, and spiritual needs, as well as your medical wishes. Newspapers have called *Five Wishes* the "living will with a heart and soul."

Five Wishes was written with the help of the American Bar Association's Commission on Law and Aging and the nation's leading experts in end-of-life care. *Five Wishes* eliminates the guesswork and spells out for your doctors and family members exactly how you wish to be treated if you become seriously ill. Because the document works so well, lawyers, doctors, hospitals and hospices, faith communities, employers, and retiree groups are making it available across the country; and more than nineteen million people of all ages have already used it (I am one of them).

If you prefer to use *Five Wishes* instead of the other documents mentioned above, destroy all copies of your old living will or durable power of attorney for healthcare. Then all you need to do is fill out and sign the form as directed. Once signed, the *Five Wishes* eliminates any advance directives you had before. Or you can write "revoked" in large letters across the copies you have. Inform your lawyer, your healthcare agent, family members, and doctor that you have filled out a *Five Wishes*.

The *Five Wishes:*

- *Wish #1: My Wish for the Person I Choose as My Healthcare Agent*
  Choose someone who knows you very well, cares about you, can make difficult decisions, and is able to stand up for you so that your wishes are followed.

- *Wish #2: My Wish for the Kind of Medical Treatment I Want or Don't Want* Your life is precious, and you deserve to be treated with dignity. When the time comes that you are very sick and unable to speak for yourself, you want the following wishes (listed below), and any other directions you have given to your healthcare agent to be respected and followed.

The next three wishes deal with personal, spiritual, and emotional desires:

- *Wish # 3: My Wish for How I Want to be Kept Comfortable* (list of desires; you will cross out anything that you don't agree with)
- *Wish # 4: My Wish for How I Want People to Treat Me* (list of desires; you will cross out anything that you don't agree with)
- *Wish #5: My Wish for What I Want My Loved Ones to Know* (list of statements; you will cross out anything that you don't agree with)
- Not part of the five wishes but how I hope to be remembered (Here is the way I filled out this section: "*She recognized and nurtured talent in others and helped many writers achieve their publishing goals.*")

What to Do Next

Give your doctor a copy of your *Five Wishes*. Be sure he or she understands your desires, is willing to follow them, and puts them in your medical record. If you are admitted to a hospital or nursing home, take a copy of *Five Wishes* with you. Keep a list of those to whom you have given copies. To order *Five Wishes,* call (888) 5-WISHES or (888) 594-7437, or go online to www.agingwithdignity.org.

If you find these official, legally binding documents intimidating or difficult to fill out at this time of your life, here are some resources you can turn to:

- Of course, if you have **a spouse, a partner, or adult children,** you can turn to one of them for assistance. Chances are, they will ask you questions about all of the topics mentioned in the *Five Wishes*:

Who is the person you trust to speak on your behalf? Who do you want to have your property after you're gone? How do you wish to be treated if you are in severe pain? What are your preferences regarding being kept alive no matter what it takes, or do you want to sign a do-not-resuscitate form?

- In the event that you do not have family to turn to, you may ask a friend or a member of your healthcare team, such as the case manager who is coordinating your care in the hospital or hospice. There are a number of organizations that provide pro bono or discounted services for senior citizens. Following is a list of legal resources (excerpted from SavvySenior.org by Jim Miller, a contributor to the *NBC Today Show* and author of *The Savvy Senior Book*):

  » **Legal Aid:** Directed by the Legal Services Corporation, legal aid offers free legal assistance to low-income people of all ages. See www.lsc.gov/find-legal-aid to locate a program in your area.

  » **Pro Bono Programs:** Usually sponsored by state or local bar associations, these programs help low-income people find volunteer lawyers who are willing to handle their cases for free. Look for a pro bono program through the American Bar Association at www.findlegalhelp.org, or through www.lawhelp.org.

  » **Senior Legal Hotlines:** There are a number of states that offer senior legal hotlines, where all seniors over age sixty have access to free legal advice over the telephone. To find the states that offer this service and their toll-free numbers, visit www.legalhotlines.org.

  » **Senior Legal Services:** Coordinated by the Administration on Aging, this service may offer free or low-cost legal advice, legal assistance, or access to legal representation to people over the age of sixty. Call the Eldercare Locator at 800-677-1116 to get your local number.

  » **National Disability Rights Network:** This is a nonprofit membership organization that provides legal assistance to people with disabilities through their Protection and Advocacy System and

Client Assistance Program. Visit www.ndrn.org to find help in your state.

- **Other Options**
  - » You could contact your state or local bar association, which may be able to refer you to a low-fee lawyer. Many bar associations offer public-service-oriented lawyer referral services. To contact your state or local bar association, visit www.americanbar.org.
  - » If you are an AARP member, you may find help at AARP's Legal Services Network from Allstate. This service provides members with a free legal consultation (up to forty-five minutes) with an attorney along with 20 percent discounts on other legal services you may need. To locate a lawyer near you, call 866-330-0753.
- Also try:
  - » **The American Bar Association (ABA)**, founded in 1878, is a voluntary bar association of lawyers and law students, which is not specific to any jurisdiction in the United States.
  - » **The National Bar Association (NBA)** was founded in 1925 and is the nation's oldest and largest national network of predominantly African-American attorneys and judges (www.nationalbar.org).

Despite our cultural aversion to thinking about death and dying, deep down, we know this is an inevitable part of life. Denial is not a good long-term strategy, but at the same time, neither is focusing on the subject obsessively. This chapter and the one about talking to your adult children cover the topic as candidly and gently as possible. For my own peace of mind, I have read what I could find on the subject, especially about how other societies deal with death. I have borrowed what resonated with me and thought about this last chapter of my life with an open mind. I think that is a better approach for me than pretending I will live forever.

Felicia Graber
From Hidden Child to Woman of Valor

Felicia Graber survived World War II by hiding in her native Poland and later fled to Western Europe. She immigrated to the United States with her husband, where she earned two college degrees. She also raised two children, taught school, and became a speaker and writer about the Holocaust, as well as a volunteer and leader in the St. Louis Jewish community. Her first book, Amazing Journey: Metamorphosis of a Hidden Child, *has been hailed as a feminist Holocaust memoir and a compelling coming-of-age story. With her brother, Dr. Leon Bialecki, she also published her father's transcribed oral history,* Our Father's Voice, a Holocaust Memoir.

◆ ◆ ◆

I am not uncomfortable talking about my end-of-life wishes and dying. In fact, I initiated the conversations with my family. I did a lot of reading about things you need to do to help your family after you pass on. After my husband, Howard, became ill, I had to prepare for the worst. I talked to my kids. I don't really know how they felt. They seemed a little nervous at first but, like I, they had to face reality. There really was no negative reaction on their part. I did most of the talking. I asked them what they wanted as far as personal inheritance items, and they each gave me a list. I also asked some of my grandchildren what they wanted.

It may be surprising, but I don't think my faith influences my attitude about death. I don't think about it from a religious point of view. I don't know what will happen, but I think I will just go to sleep.

Howard and I have all the required legal documents in place—a will, a living will, and a durable power of attorney for healthcare. We also have two documents required by Jewish law. One is a *halachic document*, which states that we donate half of our worth to our daughter before we die. The other document is a religious living will, which designates our son and a rabbi to make important medical decisions. We filled out these forms a long time ago with an attorney's help. I don't remember being upset or finding it difficult. Actually, I felt very comfortable talking to the attorney and having Howard there with me. I have given my kids all the information they might need. I wrote them a letter with legal information, how to get into my computer, my passwords, and contacts. A copy of everything is in a binder, which I update once a year.

I am leaving the more difficult medical decisions in the hands of people I trust: our son, Steven, and a rabbi. I have not indicated any instructions about a funeral, which will be a standard Orthodox ceremony. We will not be cremated, as it is against Jewish law.

My main concern is about which of us will go first. If I go first, I worry about what will happen to Howard. He will need help. We do have nursing home insurance, which includes home healthcare. I showed it to a number of people, including financial planners, who have said it's a very good policy. Their advice has been, "Don't cancel it."

I want all of our property divided between our two children. If there is anything left over beyond a specified dollar amount, we want some of it to go to the grandchildren. I have also left instructions that, when a younger grandchild gets married or earns a degree after we are gone, he or she is to receive a gift. It will be the same kind of gift their siblings received during our lifetime. I have also already given away a lot of jewelry and other personal items.

At the end of my life, if I am in pain, I would like to be made as comfortable as possible. As of now, I have had no major surgeries. I was supposed to have a knee replacement, but since we are in the midst of a pandemic, I don't know what I'm going to do about that. The knee is least of my problems. I also have issues with my back and my shoulders. I was going to hire someone to help around the house. I have spent time researching doctors, asking people questions, and reading reviews. I am a candidate for knee surgery now, although I may not be later. It's a difficult decision to make at this time during the pandemic, and I'm not sure I'm going to do it. I am very aware of being eighty.

Besides my aches and pains, I am in relatively good health. One of my problems is taking care of Howard. He has really gone downhill. He takes care of himself but has a hard time doing anything else or focusing. I do have once-a-week help, but this is an emotional time for me. It is hard to see how much he has deteriorated.

If I am at the end, do I want to be kept alive? I am leaving that up to the rabbi. That is the whole purpose of having someone make the decision for you. I did not sign a Do Not Resuscitate (DNR) form.

I had planned to get all of my writings together in a binder to give to my grandchildren, but at the moment, I feel emotionally drained. I can't seem to get myself together to do anything. On the other hand, I did just conduct a virtual meeting of our Baltimore survivors' group and gave a presentation on Zoom for a group in Israel. Perhaps I can motivate myself to do this writing project I've been putting off.

Barbara (Bobbi) Florio Graham
Author, Book Shepherd, Freelance Writer

Barbara Florio Graham is an award-winning author, publishing consultant, and marketing strategist. She is the author of three books, as well as a contributing writer to magazines, newspapers, and websites in forty-nine countries. "My Kick the Bucket List" was originally published in the Canadian magazine 55 Plus Lifestyle *and* Latin Magazine, *produced by The Latin School of Chicago. Her website was created for her famous cat, Simon Teakettle (www. simonteakettle.com), who was featured on Animal Planet TV, several CBC radio programs, and in magazines, including* Business Week. *When I asked to interview her, she sent me her "Kick the Bucket List." I didn't change a word. Bobbi is an online colleague who lives in Canada. Still writing at eighty-five, she epitomizes what it means to age with grace.*

◆ ◆ ◆

I never had a bucket list. As I think back, I realize there were several things that could have qualified.

- I rode an elephant.
- I played *12th Street Rag* in a piano and organ duet with my late mother.
- I visited the remote Canadian Sandy Lake First Nation in 1975, staying in a house with no electricity or running water, at a time when non-native visitors stayed at the nursing station.
- That visit cemented my relationship with the entire extended Meekis family, which continues forty years later.
- And I never dreamed an old friend's bucket list would lead him to finally find me, after a long search, fifty years after we were last in touch. He was my first true love, and although we live 3,000 miles apart and neither of us is well enough to travel, he phones every month and stays in touch via email.

But now that I'm over eighty, I have a Kick the Bucket List:
- Stop feeling bad about being divorced. My marriage failed; I didn't.
- Ignore TV commercials promising to erase lines, whittle my waist, or transform me in any other way so I no longer look my age. It took me a long time to learn to accept my flaws, which reveal who I really am and how I've lived.
- Don't criticize kids for dressing and speaking as if they have no respect for themselves or others. They may not have strict parents like I had, or teachers who set high standards, as I did.
- Boycott bottled water.
- Try to manage with my 20-amp electric furnace operating on just 15 amps, remembering that I'm getting by with 25 percent less energy as well.

- Accept that I used to be five-foot-two, but now I'm barely five feet. Clearly, life is grinding me down.
- Avoid high heels, Spanx, and anything that zips up the back.
- Stop mourning the cat who died too soon, and hug the new little rescue sharing my life.
- Give away my recipe collection.
- Resign myself to having thin, sparse hair and no longer wasting money on volumizing shampoos, conditioners and other treatments. If men aren't ashamed to appear in public with very little hair, why should women?
- Try not to start the Class Notes column I write for the *Barnard Alumnae Magazine* with another death announcement.
- Refrain from the tendency of those who live alone to ignore holidays and special occasions. Buy the kind of special treats I'd enjoy if I were invited to a posh party, put on a favorite but comfortable outfit and jewelry I still love too much to give away, and watch movies I've saved for those occasions.
- Don't save favorite treats for special days. As Jacques Torres said, "Life is short; eat dessert first."
- Refuse any recommended procedures ending with "opsy" or "oscopy."
- Don't complain about things nobody else can do anything about. If something is leaking, broken, making an annoying noise, or not working properly, find someone who actually has the ability to fix it. But keep in mind that some minor things are not calamities, and we just have to put up with them.
- Remember that there's no shame in asking for what you want, but that doesn't mean others will always comply. Understand that sometimes their failure to respond has nothing to do with me, just with their busy lives.
- Put things into perspective. Of course, I can't do what I used to do. That isn't a tragedy; it's the price we pay for not dying young.

- Caution my loved ones not to put me on life support unless there's a good chance I can recover sufficiently to enjoy a meal and conversation with friends. Remember when Joan Rivers said she no longer wanted to remain alive unless she could still stand on a stage and be funny.
- Avoid people who make simple things difficult, and difficult things impossible.
- Don't forget to appreciate connections I have with former students, including one who sends me birthday gifts every year; a high school friend, just a year younger who still bicycles everywhere; and a writing colleague who bought a goat for a boy in Kenya to honor me on my 80th birthday.
- Disagree with Toni Morrison, who announced recently that there are only three things left to say: "No." "Shut Up." "Get Out."

As I follow my Kick the Bucket List, I want to remember to keep saying "Yes ... Tell me more ... and Come in."

© *Barbara Florio Graham, used with permission*

RESOURCES

Alexander, Anne. *That Sugar Smart Diet: Stop Craving and Lose Weight While Still Enjoying This Sweet Tea Love!* Pennsylvania: Rodale Books. 2013.

Appleton, Nancy. *Stopping Inflammation: Relieving the Cause of Degenerative Diseases.* New York: Square One Publishers. 2005.

Appleton, Nancy. *Suicide by Sugar.* New York: Square One Publishers. 2009.

Bernhard, Toni. *How to Be Sick: A Buddhist-Inspired Guide for the Chronically Ill and Their Caregivers.* Massachusetts: Wisdom Publications. 2010.

Bloomfield, Harold H., Robert K. Cooper, PhD, John Gray. *Think Safe, Be Safe: The Only Guide to Inner Peace and Outer Security.* New York: Three Rivers Press. 1998.

Bridges, William. *Transitions: Making Sense of Life's Changes.* New York: Hachette Book Group. 2019.

Buettner, Dan. *The Blue Zones, Second Addition: Nine Lessons for Living Longer from the People Who've Lived the Longest.* Washington, DC: National Geographic. 2012.

Burns, David D. *Feeling Good: The New Mood Therapy*. New York: HarperCollins Publishers. 1998.

Case, Bill. *Stand tall, Don't Fall: Improve Your Posture, Balance, and Strength*. Nevada: ChickLit Media Group. 2017.

Collard, Patrizia. *The Little Book of Mindfulness: 10 Minutes a Day to Less Stress, More Peace*. London: Octopus Publishing Group. 2014.

Esty, PhD, Katharine. *Eightysomethings: A Practical Guide to Letting Go, Aging Well, and Finding Unexpected Happiness*. New York: Skyhorse. 2019.

Fejetem, Michael. *Strength Training for Seniors: How to Rewind Your Biological Clock*. California: Hunter House. 2006.

Ferrin, Kelly. *What's Age Got to Do with It—Secrets of Aging in Extraordinary Ways*. Oklahoma: Red Zone Publishing. 2004.

Forem, Jack. *Transcendental Meditation*. California: Hay House. 1973.

Gawande, Atul. *Being Mortal: Medicine and What Matters in the End*. New York: Henry Holt and Company. 2017.

Koyama, Ruthanne. *Staying Home in Your 70s, 80s, and Beyond: A Practical Guide to Staying in Your Own Home*. Independently Published. 2015.

Marantz Henig, Robin. *How a Woman Ages—Growing Older: What to Expect and What You Can Do About It*. New York: Ballantine/Esquire Press. 1985.

Matthews, Jessica. *Stretching to Stay Young: Simple Workouts to Keep You Flexible, Energized, and Pain Free*. California: Althea Press. 2016.

Metzl, Jordan. *The Exercise Cure: The Doctors All Natural, No-Pill Prescription for Better Health in Longer Life.* Pennsylvania: Rodale Books. 2013.

Nelson, Miriam E., PhD. *Strong Women Stay Young.* New York: Bantam Books. 1998.

Nuland, Sherwin B. *The Art of Aging: A Doctor's Prescription for Well-Being.* New York: The Random House Publishing Group. 2007.

O'Neill, Dr. Barbara and CFP®, Jane White. *Financial Fitness for the Rest of Your Life: What Older Adults Need to Know About Money.* New Jersey: New Jersey Coalition for Financial Education. 2019.

Passanisi, Kathleen Keller. *It's your life—Choose well.* Missouri: Movere Publishing. 2003.

Perlmutter, David. *Grain Brain: The Surprising Truth About Wheat, Carbs, and Sugar—Your Brain's Silent Killers.* New York: Little, Brown and Company. 2013.

Pipher, Mary. *Women Rowing North: Navigating Life's Currents and Flourishing as We Age.* New York: Bloomsbury Publishing. 2020.

Ratey MD, John and Eric Hagerman. *Spark: The Revolutionary New Science of Exercise and the Brain.* New York: Little, Brown and Company. 2013.

Richardson, Corinne. *Coping While Hoping for Better Health: Facing the Challenges of a Disease.* Missouri: Willcott & Corn Books. 2014.

Roberts RN, Kasia. *Anti-inflammatory Diet: Your Ultimate Guide to Healing Inflammation, Alleviating Pain and Slowing Aging.* Toronto: The Fruitful Mind. 2015.

Shepherd, Sue. *The Complete FODMAP Diet: A Revolutionary Plan for Managing IBS and Other Digestive Disorders.* New York: The Experiment. 2013.

Steinem, Gloria. *Doing Sixty & Seventy.* California/Australia: Eldership Academy Press. 2006.

Viorst, Judith, and Laura Gibson. *I'm Too Young to Be Seventy: And Other Delusions.* New York: Simon & Schuster. 2005.

Viorst, Judith. *Unexpectedly Eighty: And Other Adaptations.* New York: Simon & Schuster. 2010.

Weil, Andrew, MD. *Healthy Aging: A Lifelong Guide Your Well-Being.* New York: Knopf Doubleday Publishing Group. 2008.

Wheat Belly: Lose the Wheat, Lose the Weight, and Find Your Path Back to Health. Pennsylvania: Rodale Books. 2019.

ABOUT THE AUTHOR

Bobbi Linkemer is a writing coach, ghostwriter, and editor who retired in 2019 at the age of eighty-two. During her fifty-year career, she has written for a wide range of publications and businesses. She is the author of twenty-seven books and has helped many aspiring authors write and publish their books. Bobbi's interest in aging is personal because she is an older adult and practical because she is aware of the many available options to help her get the most out of life.

She continues to contribute to her community, encourage and mentor aspiring authors, and help older adults maintain their health and vitality throughout their lives.

Dear Reader,

Thank you so much for reading *How to Age with Grace*. I hope you will find it a helpful guide to living your best life now and in the years to come. **Your feedback is important to me, so I hope you will take a few minutes to write a brief review on Amazon.** Also, please visit HowtoAgewithGrace.com and leave a comment, email me at bobbi@howtoagewithgrace.com, or give me a call at 314-495-8589. I'd love to hear from you.

CPSIA information can be obtained
at www.ICGtesting.com
Printed in the USA
LVHW081551271021
701603LV00013BA/2078